P9-EMH-890

Allergic Diseases in Children

The Science, the Superstition and the Stories

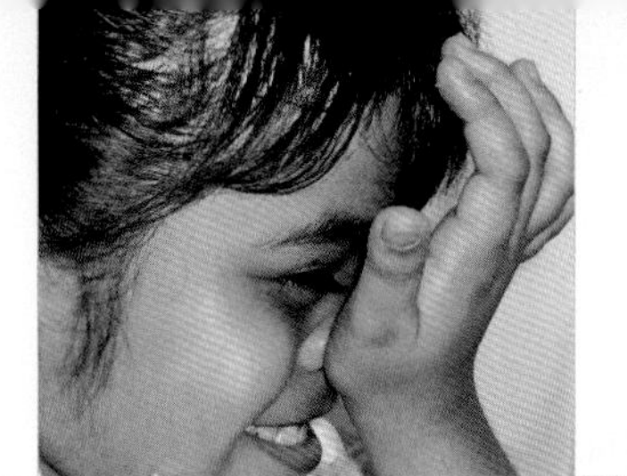

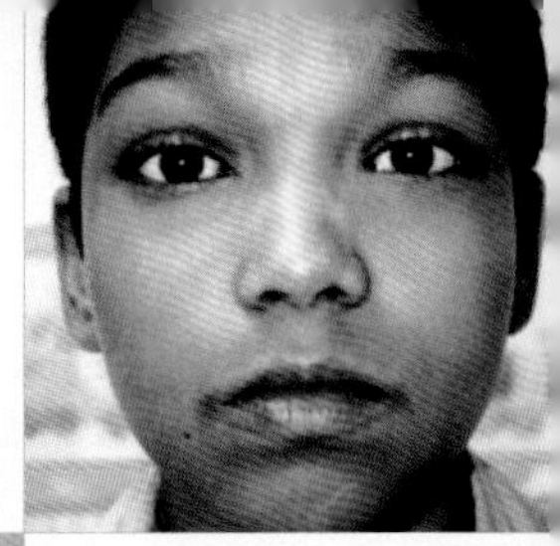

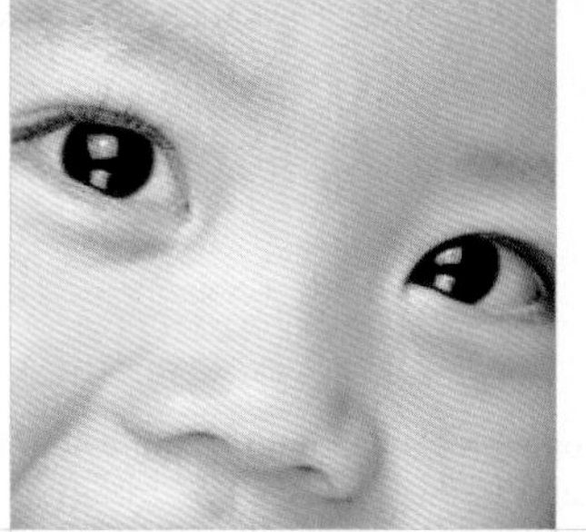

Hugo Van Bever

Allergic Diseases in Children

The Science, the Superstition and the Stories

World Scientific

NEW JERSEY • LONDON • SINGAPORE • BEIJING • SHANGHAI • HONG KONG • TAIPEI • CHENNAI

Published by

World Scientific Publishing Co. Pte. Ltd.
5 Toh Tuck Link, Singapore 596224
USA office: 27 Warren Street, Suite 401-402, Hackensack, NJ 07601
UK office: 57 Shelton Street, Covent Garden, London WC2H 9HE

Library of Congress Cataloging-in-Publication Data
Van Bever, Hugo.
Allergic diseases in children : the science, the superstition and the stories / Hugo Van Bever.
p. cm.
Includes index.
ISBN-13: 978-981-4273-53-4 (hardcover : alk. paper)
ISBN-10: 981-4273-53-8 (hardcover : alk. paper)
1. Allergy in children. I. Title.
RJ386.V36 2009
618.92'97--dc22

2009015202

British Library Cataloguing-in-Publication Data
A catalogue record for this book is available from the British Library.

Design by **LAB Creations** (A Unit of World Scientific Publishing Co. Pte. Ltd.)

Printed in Singapore by Mainland Press Pte Ltd.

Foreword

Allergic diseases are of increasing prevalence around the world. There is also evidence of significant morbidity from this group of conditions. Despite its relatively common occurrence, there is still a significant lack of understanding of the cause(s), its management and even more so the prognosis and also prevention of these diseases. This applies not only to parents, the general public but also healthcare workers. It is very timely that a book encapsulating the spectrum of facts relevant to the understanding and appreciation of allergies in childhood is written. This is even more beneficial and useful when it encompasses the local cultural and traditional beliefs that significantly impact on its management.

Professor Hugo Van Bever has been in clinical practice in pediatric allergy for more than 25 years, spending more than 15 years in Europe and more recently 7 years in Singapore. With a deep appreciation of the clinical issues in childhood allergy and having personally been involved in teaching and research in this field, Professor Hugo is the most aptly qualified to pen such a book. He has also been an active member of "I CAN !" (The Children's Asthma and Allergy Network) at the University Children's Medical Institute (UCMI) of the National

University Hospital, Singapore. The program emphasizes asthma and allergy education, facilitating and encouraging every child with asthma and allergies to lead a totally normal and active lifestyle despite the conditions. This book is very much an extension of this program, dedicated to the parents, caregivers and anyone who cares to know more about asthma and allergies in childhood and who is committed to helping these children lead an unrestricted fruitful life.

I am very pleased and proud that the pediatric services in NUH continues to contribute to patient care and education in practical ways that enhance the quality of life of our young patients and their families. I am certain that this book will be an important tool for every parent and even healthcare workers and an indispensible guide for every medical student alike.

I congratulate Professor Hugo on this achievement and you, the reader, for making the right choice to further your understanding of asthma and allergies. I wish you many hours of fruitful learning and more importantly application of this knowledge for the good of the very people it is meant to benefit – our young ones with asthma and allergies in Singapore and the region and beyond.

Associate Professor Daniel Goh
Chief of Paediatrics
University Children's Medical Institute
National University Hospital
And
Pioneering Chair of the Children's
Asthma and Allergy Network
("I CAN" Programme)
National University Hospital
Singapore

Acknowledgements

This book would never have been written without the help of many people. Actually, so many people helped me through the years that it became impossible to sum them all up. Therefore, now and here (using the *cliché*): sincere apologies to all those whom I might have forgotten to mention. I am sure you will forgive me!

I wish to thank all those allergic children, their parents and their families who inspired me stimulate my desire to continue to seek new knowledge, and to keep looking for causes and treatments, and to never give up in clinical research. It was their allergic problems that kept me going during the past twenty-five years (and I hope more years of research and commitment to come).

I am grateful to my colleagues ("boss" Daniel, Lynette, Bee Wah, Kay Yan, Irvin and all the others) at NUS and NUH for their help and the opportunities they gave me: the discussions held, opinions shared, and great support rendered during clinical work. Also, thanks to my colleagues at the National Skin Centre (especially Giam Yoke) for their assistance and for providing me with fantastic pictures on skin allergic problems.

I wish also to thank my colleagues and friends worldwide — Peter Soemantri, Ruby Pawankar, Gideon Lack, Peter

Smith, Pakit Vichyanond, John Warner, Ulrich Wahn, and many others whose names I will start to recall as this book goes into printing. Thanks for teaching me and supporting me; thanks for disagreeing with me and debating with me; thanks for sending me pictures of allergic children, and for hanging out with me during all those international congresses.

I wish to acknowledge the pharmaceutical companies - Abbott Laboratoties, Schering-Plough, Merck Sharp & Dohme, AstraZeneca, and UCB - who have made the printing of this book possible and who gave me total freedom (and no double-checking!) in the writing of this book. Thanks guys!

Thanks to Sook-Cheng Lim (World Scientific) and to Runzi Zhang (with her cute baby William) (Delphin Singapore) for their support and guidance during the writing – reading – rewriting – rereading, etc... Thanks Sook for taking a chance and putting the edition in your hands. Thanks Runzi for your enthusiasm (and switching off your HP from time to time).

Thanks to all my "non-medical" friends ("Punnut, Linda, Lilly, Danny, Vic *et les autres*...") for their support and understanding. You guys know me, you knew when to leave me alone, when to ask me out, when to call me and - more important - when not to call me. Thanks Punnut for your inspiration, and for all those "Einstein-like" talks (at least we tried) on the meaning of life, religion (Buddhism), helping people, helping children and on the aim of knowledge and science. I am sure that one day you will write your own book too! (... and I agree that LV-bags are nice, but they will never be the mirror of the quality of the brain).

Thanks to my fantastic family members for support, freedom, understanding and love. I dedicate this book to my mom ("mom, you're the best") to Hilde, Stijn, Eva, Bart, Lorin, Sam and Ilse, to my only auntie "Tante Monie" who inspired me when I was a child and to all the allergic and non-allergic children in the world.

... All of you have shown me what the meaning of life should be: be useful, passionate, down to earth and don't forget that money is as evident as oxygen: for everybody, and free of charge!

Hugo Van Bever
Singapore, May 2009

About the Author

Hugo PS Van Bever completed his medical studies at the State University of Ghent, Belgium (1971–1978) and did his training in pediatrics at the Children's Hospital, State University of Ghent, Belgium from 1978–1983. Following that he became Resident in Paediatric Allergy and Pulmonology, at the University of Antwerp, Belgium from 1984–1993. He was appointed as Associate Professor in Paediatric Allergy and Pulmonology, from 1993–1997 and as Professor in Paediatric Allergy and Pulmonology, University of Antwerp, Belgium from 1997. From 1997–2001, he was also the Head of the Department of Paediatrics, University of Antwerp, Belgium.

He joined the National University Singapore as Professor and Senior Consultant in Paediatric Allergy and Immunology at the Department of Paediatrics in June 2002. In On 28–30 November 2003, he organized an international Asian Pacific Association of Paediatric Allergy, Respirology and Immunology workshop, held from 28–30 November, in Singapore, entitled "Asthma and Allergies in Young Children in South-East Asia." He is now an active member of the board of APAPARI, in which he is responsible for research and education in paediatric allergy.

Hugo van Bever MD, PhD

Professor in Paediatrics
Department of Paediatrics
National University Hospital/
National University of Singapore
Yong Loo Lin School of Medicine,
National University of Singapore

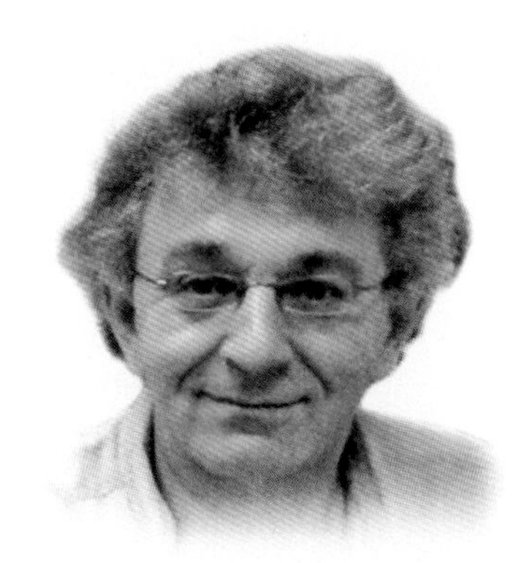

He attended two NUS-Harvard Medical International Programs for Educators in October 2005 and October 2006, respectively.

He has been Associate Editor of the European Respiratory Journal (1993–1998). Currently, he is member of the Editorial Board of Pediatric Allergy and Immunology and is the Editor-in-Chief of the Journal of Allergy. He is a reviewer for the European Journal of Paediatrics, Pediatrics, Paediatric Allergy and Immunology, Allergy, Paediatric Pulmonology, the European Respiratory Journal, Paediatric Research, British Medical Journal, the American Journal of Respiratory and Critical Care Medicine and Archives Diseases of Childhood.

Hugo Van Bever defended his PhD thesis successfully in June 1993 at the University of Antwerp. The title of this thesis is: "Late asthmatic reactions in childhood asthma and influence of specific immunotherapy upon the late asthmatic reaction."

He has published more than 300 papers in national and international journals. His main research interest areas are pediatric allergy, pediatric asthma and pediatric respiratory infections. His current research is focused on eczema, allergic rhinitis, sublingual immunotherapy and food allergy.

Content

	Foreword	vi
	Acknowledgments	viii
	About the Author	x
	General Introduction	xiv
Chapter 1	On Allergy and Allergic Reactions	2
Chapter 2	Epidemiology of Allergic Diseases in Asia	32
Chapter 3	The Allergens	44
Chapter 4	Asthma in Children	72
Chapter 5	Allergy of Upper Airways — Allergic rhinitis, Allergic rhino-sinusitis and Allergic conjunctivitis	92
Chapter 6	Eczema or Atopic Dermatitis	110
Chapter 7	Urticaria and Angioedema	140
Chapter 8	Food Allergy	156
Chapter 9	Drug Allergy	186
Chapter 10	Severe Allergic Reactions: What Can We Do?	212
Chapter 11	Diagnosis and Management of Allergic Diseases	226
Chapter 12	General Conclusion — The Future of Allergic Diseases in Children	262
	Common Questions Asked by Parents on Allergy	268
	References	272
	Index	288

General Introduction

Allergic diseases have become the most common group of diseases in children, affecting more than 20% of children worldwide. During the last three decades there has been a tremendous increase in allergy disorders in children, mainly in the developed countries (Fig. 1). Allergic diseases are a growing health problem across the world.

The increase in allergic diseases can be attributed to adoption of a Western lifestyle: It is the price we have to pay when we reach a higher standard of living (Fig. 2). In general, it can be stated that the wealthier a country is, the more commonly allergy will occur among its children.

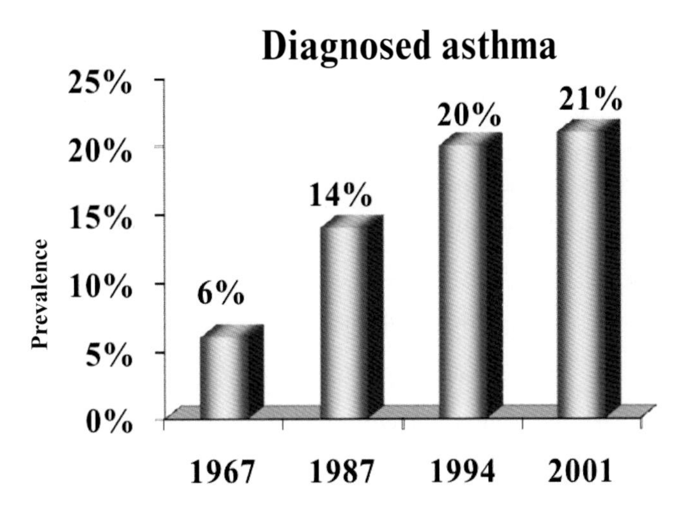

Fig. 1 The increase in incidence of asthma in Singapore from 1967 to 2001. (from: Wang and co-worbers, *Arch Dis Child* (2004) **89**:423.)

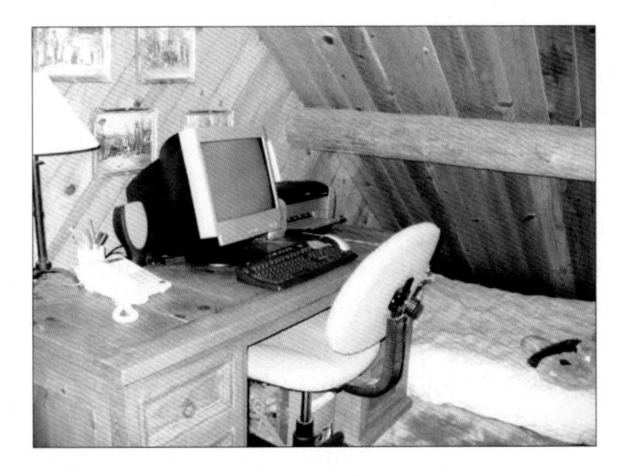

Fig. 2 A modern child's bedroom contains more than a bed. Most children have their own television set and computer, spending more time in the bedroom.

Table 1 Inheritance of Allergy

Parents	Risk for children
1. both are non-allergic	15 – 20%
2. only father is allergic	40%
3. only mother is allergic	50%
4. both are allergic	70%
5. both are very allergic	> 90%

For most people with an allergic disease, allergy would first appear during infancy or childhood. It is not surprising, then, that allergic disorders rank first among children's chronic diseases.

Any child can become allergic, but children from families with a history of allergy are more likely to become allergic. Children may inherit the tendency to become allergic from their parents, but not all of them will develop active allergic disease (Table 1). On the other hand, children with no allergy in the family can develop symptoms of allergy. The mechanisms of inheritance are still poorly understood. One thing is for sure: inheritance of an allergy is a complex phenomenon as many modes and many types of genes are involved.

The more allergies in the parents, the higher the risk for the child to become allergic. However, even if both parents are non-allergic, there is still a 15 – 20% risk that the child will become allergic.

Allergies can show up in different ways in children. Some children develop skin rashes (eczema or hives) from allergy; others suffer from asthma and still others develop allergy of the nose (allergic rhinitis), such as hay fever (also referred to as seasonal allergic rhinitis).

Allergic rhinitis is the most common of all allergy problems, followed by asthma and eczema (Fig. 3).

Allergic rhinitis (Fig. 4) is characterized by a runny, itchy nose, sneezing, postnasal drip (dripping of phlegm in the

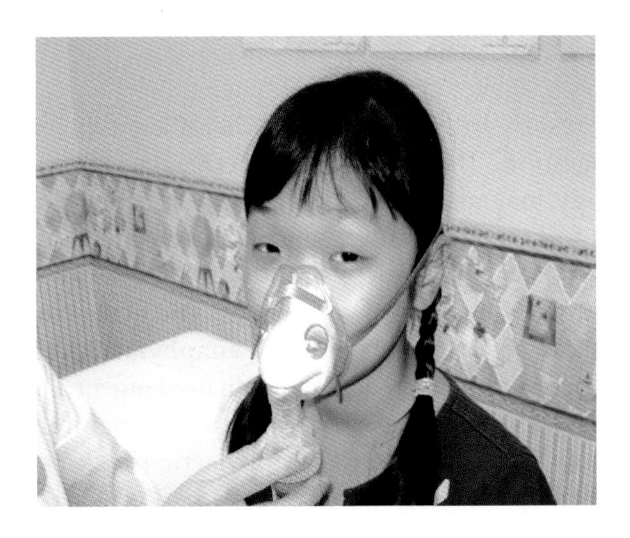

Fig. 3 Asthmatic girl treated with a nebulizer during an acute asthma attack.

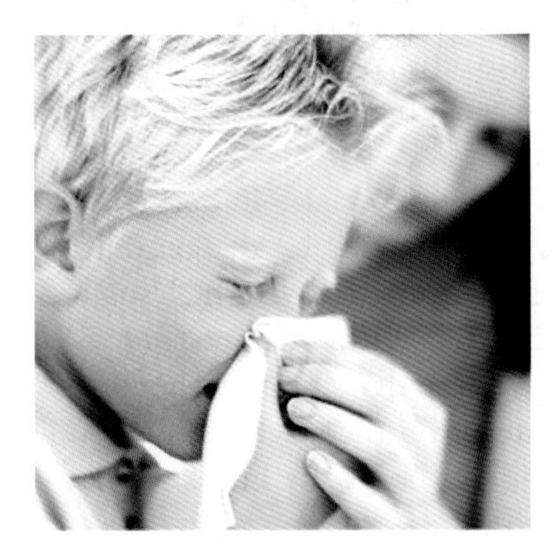

Fig. 4 A child with allergic rhinitis.

throat which results in cough) and nasal congestion. The child with this allergy may also have itchy, watery and red eyes and chronic ear problems. Allergic rhinitis can occur at any time of the year, seasonally or year-round. In most Asian countries with a tropical climate, seasonal rhinitis is extremely rare because of the lack of seasons (no pollen season in tropical countries).

Asthma is an allergic disease of the lower airways (of the bronchi). Asthma presents as attacks of shortness of breath, cough and wheezing (i.e. a whistling sound during breathing). Asthma can also present as a chronic cough. Allergy is not the only cause of asthma. In particular in young children, asthma can also be triggered by viral infection of the airways.

Eczema or atopic dermatitis is characterized by the existence of a chronic itchy rash. Usually children with eczema (Fig. 5) have very dry skin and show red patches on the face, neck, elbow folds, back of the knees, ankles and wrists.

Other allergic manifestations are: **urticaria** (hives) (Fig. 6), **vomiting** and **chronic diarrhea**, and **failure to thrive**. In some children, allergy can present as a severe and dangerous event, called **anaphylactic shock**. These children need urgent and intensive treatment, as manifestations of anaphylactic shock can become fatal.

The Allergens usually causing allergic symptoms are inhaled allergens that can cause the symptoms through the airways. In other cases, various different foods, such as peanuts or seafood, can be responsible for allergic symptoms.

Just remember

- Allergies are common in children and can manifest in different ways
- The most common manifestation of allergy is allergic rhinitis
- Allergy to inhalants is far more common than allergy to foods
- In tropical regions, house dust mites (Fig. 7) are the main cause of allergy

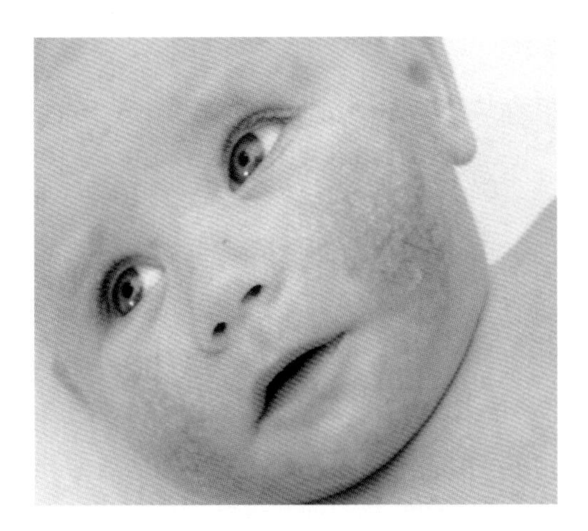

Fig. 5 A child with eczema. Baby with severe eczema in the face.

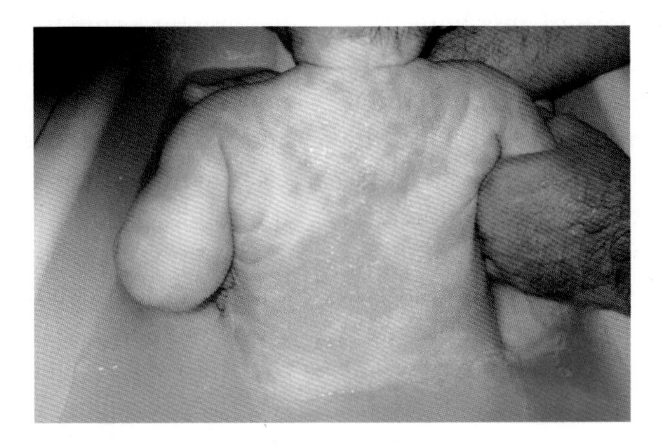

Fig. 6 Child with acute urticaria (courtesy of Prof. Peter Smith, Australia).

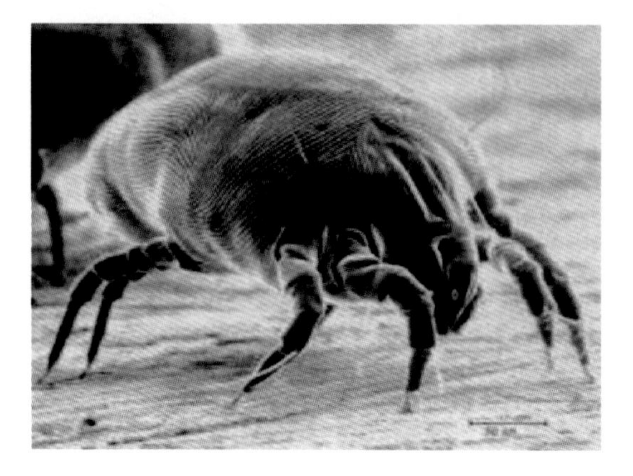

Fig. 7 House dust mite. The various different types of house dust mites are the most common cause of childhood allergies in tropical countries.

About the book

The purpose of this book is to share information and knowledge on allergic disorders in children with everybody, especially with parents of allergic children. Allergic disorders in children are a common and growing problem. From my experience, many parents lack correct information on allergy. This has led to wrong approaches in dealing with the problem, as well as false expectations and disappointment. Moreover, parents will keep looking for a cure for their child, and may end up with all kinds of non-scientifically proven testing and treatments. Sometimes these treatments can be harmful for the child.

The book comprises twelve chapters, each covering a specific aspect of allergy in children. The first part covers general issues, such as underlying mechanisms, allergens, and epidemiology of allergic diseases. In the second part, specific allergic diseases are covered. The book ends with considerations on diagnosis and treatment, and offers suggestions for future research on allergy in children. At the end, common questions on allergy are answered briefly.

I hope that this book will provide useful information to the public, especially parents of allergic children. Based on current scientific information, the book should help allergic children to obtain optimal diagnosis and treatment of their allergic disease. In case you have any questions or remarks or views, please email me on: allergyinchild@wspc.com

I will try to answer ASAP.

Hugo Van Bever

1

On Allergy and Allergic Reactions

This chapter is a general introduction and covers three aspects of childhood allergies, including a short overview on the immune system. For further reading on the immune system, the reader could refer to more specialized literature or to the Internet (see chapter on references).

- **What is allergy?**
- **What causes allergy?**
- **What are the main manifestations of allergy?**

In short, allergy is a feature, not a disease. It is due to the ability of the human body to produce IgE against harmless substances, called allergens. Allergy is a very dynamic process, especially in young children. Allergic reactions come and go: children can grow out of allergies, and new allergies can occur at any age, but the occurrence of new allergies in elderly people is very exceptional.

What is allergy?

The term allergy is used to describe an inappropriate and harmful response of the immune system to a harmless foreign substance (usually a protein), that results in an immune response that can cause symptoms and disease in a predisposed person. Allergy in itself is not a disease, nor is it a diagnosis. It is merely **a genetic feature** of the human body: people can be allergic or non-allergic. Nowadays, most people are non-allergic, but over last the three decades more and more people, especially children have become allergic.

Allergy means that the body reacts in a particular way to the environment by producing a specific type of antibody. That specific antibody, called immunoglobulin E (IgE), induces a hypersensitivity reaction of the body through activating different cell types, including mast cells (see Fig. 1). Cell activation can lead to "inflammation," which means that the body attains a state of alertness, and that in the different organs (such as the skin or the airways) swelling, redness and cell infiltration occurs. It is the inflammation that causes the symptoms. If the inflammation occurs in the skin, eczema will result. In the airways, inflammation can result in asthma (lower airways) or rhinitis (upper airways). Symptoms can also occur in other organs such as the intestine, eyes, or even the brain.

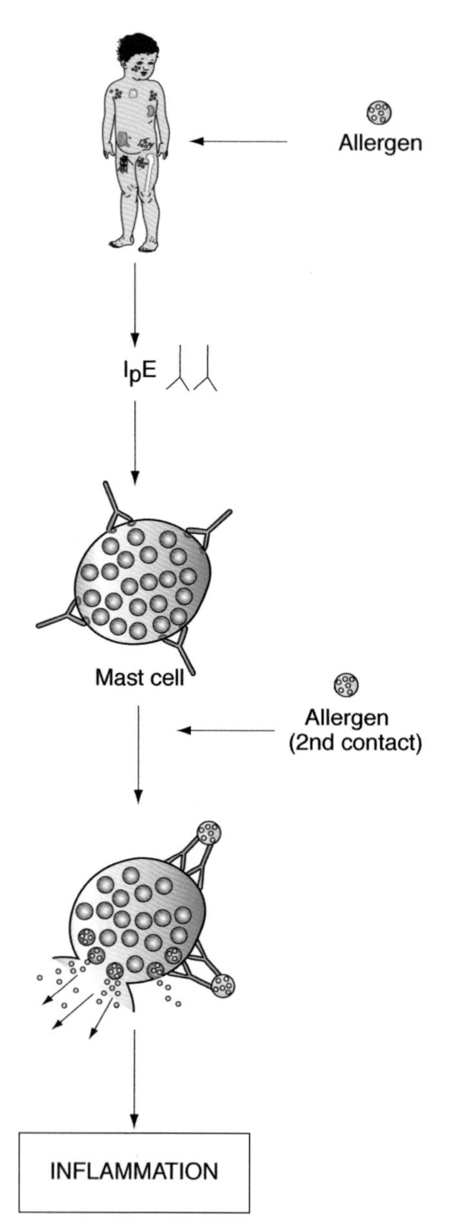

Fig. 1 Mechanism of an allergic reaction.

1. A potentially allergic child comes into contact with an allergen (through inhalation, ingestion, or through direct contact with the skin).
2. Production of immunoglobulin E (IgE) by certain types of cells (B lymphocytes). The IgE circulates in the blood, and comes into contact with different cells, tissues and organs.
3. IgE binds to mast cells via an IgE-receptor in the membrane of the mast cell.
4. A second contact with the same allergen results in destruction of the cell wall of the mast cell.
5. Different molecules are released by the mast cell. One of these many molecules is histamine.
6. Various molecules (mediators, cytokines, and others) from the mast cell induce attraction and activation of other cells, resulting in inflammation. This inflammation occurs most commonly in the nose (rhinitis), in the lungs (asthma) and in the skin (eczema).

On the Immune System

Through a process known as **the immune response**, the immune system protects us against invaders from the environment. It is composed of many types of cells that collectively protect the body from bacterial, parasitic, fungal, and viral infections. The immune system reacts to every foreign substance that we encounter in the environment, even to substances that are beneficial or totally harmless, such as food. Besides a protective function against invaders, the immune system has other functions that keep us healthy. One example is that the immune system protects us from growth of tumor cells.

White blood cells, also called leukocytes, make up the main cell type of the immune system. These cells are produced in lymphoid organs like the bone marrow, thymus and spleen and move within the body through channels that are known as lymphatic vessels.

Two major groups of white blood cells play a role in immune response: myelocytes and lymphocytes. Myelocytes, being phagocytic, engulf and chew up invading substances, while lymphocytes play several different roles in combating invaders. Lymphocytes are classified into B and T cells. B cells produce and secrete antibodies, while T cells help to destroy the invaders by regulating the function of other cells.

The lymphocytic network is a very complex network, comprising many types of lymphocytes. Schematically, it is mainly composed of two parts: one part (B cells) being responsible for the production of different types of antibodies, each with a specific role in our defence against micro-organisms (viruses, bacteria, etc); and the second part comprises different types of cells that are directly involved in protecting and defending us. This latter part is mainly built up of different T subsets of lymphocytes. These lymphocytes secrete substances that help to regulate the functions of other cells in the defence of the body. These substances are known as cytokines, lymphokines, and interleukins.

The immune system is built up and refined over millions of years. Its various different functions are carried out by different types of cells, giving rise to a lot of overlapping functions, and resulting in a very robust and reliable defence system.

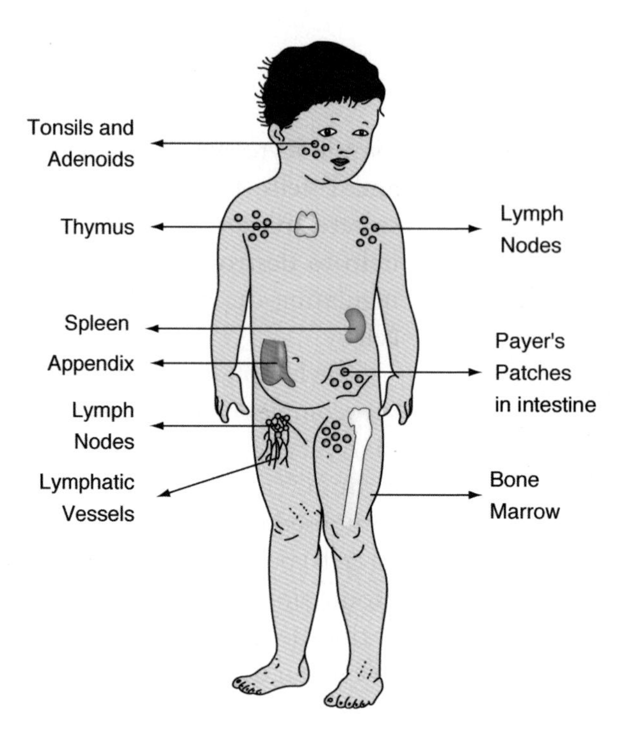

Fig. 2 Organs of the immune system.

The Organs of the Immune System (Fig. 2)

Bone Marrow — All the cells of the immune system are initially derived from the bone marrow, more specifically from bone marrow-derived stem cells. These cells differentiate into either mature cells of the immune system or into precursors of cells that migrate out of the bone marrow to continue their maturation elsewhere. Cells that are produced by the bone marrow are: B lymphocytes (which are responsible for antibody production), natural killer lymphocytes, granulocytes and immature thymocytes (that will mature in the thymus), in addition to red blood cells and platelets.

Thymus — The function of the thymus is to produce mature T lymphocytes. Through a remarkable maturation process sometimes referred to as "thymic education" T cells that are beneficial to the immune system are spared, while those T cells that might evoke a non-favorable autoimmune response are eliminated. The mature T cells are then released into the bloodstream.

Spleen — The spleen is an immunologic filter of the blood. It is made up of different types of cells, including B cells, T cells, macrophages, dendritic cells, natural killer cells and red blood cells. The main function of the spleen is to capture foreign materials (antigens) from the blood. An immune response in the spleen is initiated when the macrophage or dendritic cells present the antigen to the appropriate B or T cells. The spleen can be considered as an immunological conference center. In the spleen, B cells become activated and produce large amounts of antibodies. Also, old red blood cells are destroyed in the spleen.

Lymph Nodes — The lymph nodes function as immunologic filters and are found throughout the body. Composed mostly of T cells, B cells, dendritic cells and macrophages, the nodes drain fluid from most of our tissues. Antigens are filtered out of the lymph in the lymph nodes before the lymph returns to the circulation. In a similar fashion as the spleen, the macrophages and dendritic cells that capture antigens present these foreign materials to T and B cells, consequently initiating an immune response.

The Cells of the Immune System (Fig. 3)

1. T-Cells — T lymphocytes are usually divided into two major subsets: helper T cells (Fig. 4) and killer/suppressor T cells. The two types of cells are functionally different.

The T helper subset (Th cells), also called the $CD4^+$ T cell, is a pertinent coordinator of immune regulation. Nowadays four types of $CD4^+$ cells are distinguished: Th-1, Th-2, Th-17 and T-reg (regulatory T cells), and it is very likely that in the future further discoveries will lead to the identification of other types of T cells (Fig. 4). The main function of the T helper cell is to augment or potentiate and regulate immune responses through the secretion of specialized factors that activate other white blood cells to fight off infection. Th-1 cells are involved in normal immune responses against viruses or bacteria, while

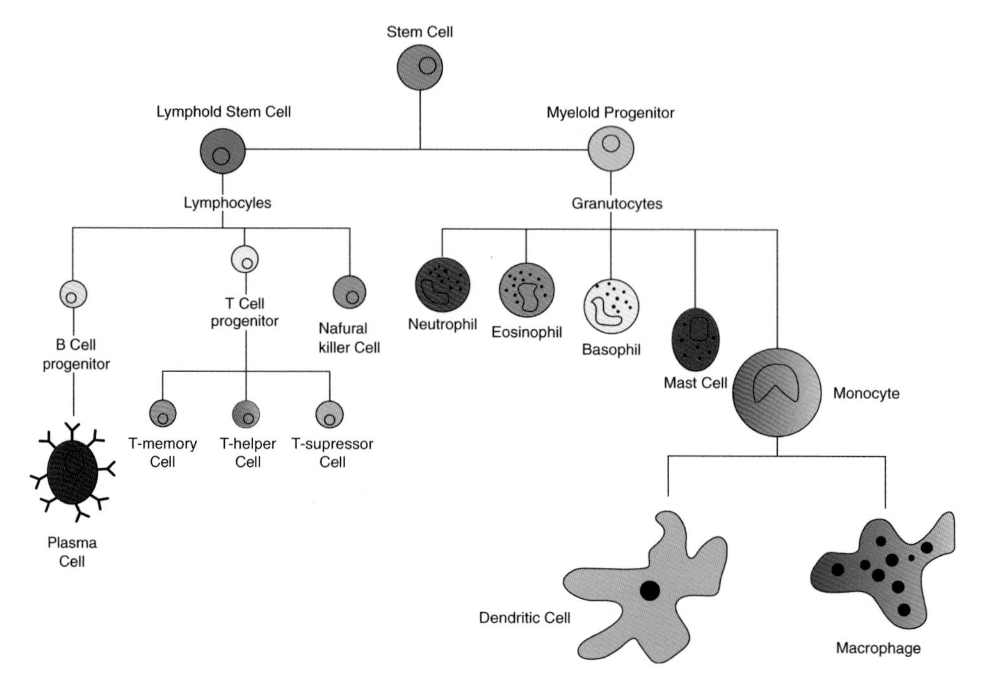

Fig. 3 Different cells of the immune system.

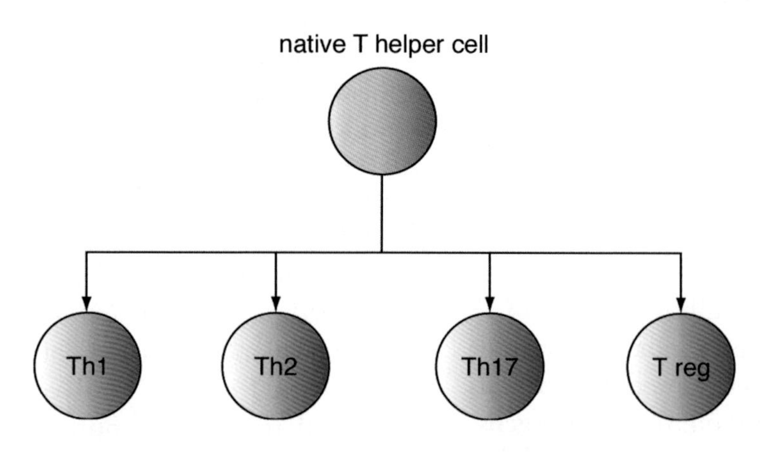

Fig. 4 The 4 major types of T helper cells (CD4$^+$ T cell).

Th-2 cells are mainly involved in allergic reactions, inducing IgE production via a number of mechanisms. Th-17 have recently been discovered and seem to be involved in a number of specific immune responses, including responses that can lead to the occurrence of eczema. T-reg cells are mainly regulating cells that are responsible for a healthy balance of immune responses throughout the body.

The second type of T cells is called the T killer/suppressor subset, also called as $CD8^+$ T cells. These cells are important in directly killing certain tumor cells, viral-infected cells and sometimes parasites. The $CD8^+$ T cells are also important in down-regulation of immune responses.

Both types of T cells can be found throughout the body. They often depend on the secondary lymphoid organs (the lymph nodes and spleen) as sites where activation occurs, but they are also found in other tissues of the body, most conspicuously the liver, lung, blood, and intestinal and reproductive tracts.

2. Natural Killer Cells — Natural killer cells, often referred to as NK cells, are similar to the killer T cell subset ($CD8^+$ T cells). They function as cells that directly kill certain tumor cells and viral-infected cells, most notably herpes and cytomegalovirus-infected cells. NK cells, unlike the $CD8^+$ (killer) T cells, kill their targets without a prior "conference" in the lymphoid organs. However, NK cells that have been activated due to secretions from $CD4^+$ T cells will kill their tumor or viral-infected targets more effectively.

3. B Cells — The major function of B lymphocytes is the production of different types of antibodies in response to foreign proteins of bacteria, viruses, and tumor cells. Antibodies are specialized proteins that specifically recognize and bind to one particular protein (i.e. antigen or allergen). Antibody production and binding to a foreign substance or antigen, often is critical as a means of signaling other cells to engulf, kill or remove that substance from the body.

4. Granulocytes or Polymorphonuclear (PMN) Leukocytes — Another group of white blood cells is collectively referred to as granulocytes or polymorphonuclear leukocytes (PMNs). Granulocytes are composed of three types of

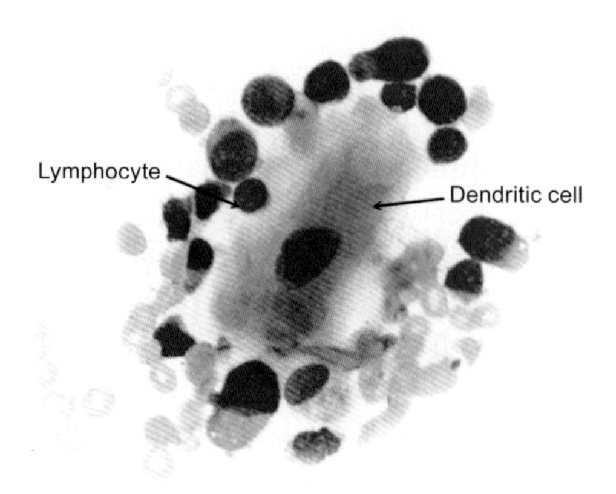

Fig. 5 Dendritic cells act as antigen-presenting cells, and are involved in the initiation of immune response, by presenting the allergens to the T lymphocyte compartment of the immune system.

cells identified as neutrophils, eosinophils and basophiles, based on their staining characteristics with certain dyes, under the microscope. These cells are predominantly important in the removal of bacteria and parasites from the body. They engulf these foreign bodies and degrade them using their powerful enzymes. Eosinophils are involved in allergic reactions, and also in defence against parasites. Basophiles have a number of functions, and are also involved in the initial phase of an allergic reaction.

5. Macrophages — Macrophages are important in the regulation of immune responses. They are often referred to as scavengers or antigen-presenting cells (APC) because they pick up and ingest foreign materials and present these antigens to other cells of the immune system such as T cells and B cells.

6. Dendritic Cells (Fig. 5) — Another cell type, addressed only recently, is the dendritic cell. Dendritic cells, which also originate in the bone marrow, function as antigen presenting cells (APC) and can be considered as a type of macrophage. In fact, the dendritic cells are more efficient APCs than macrophages.

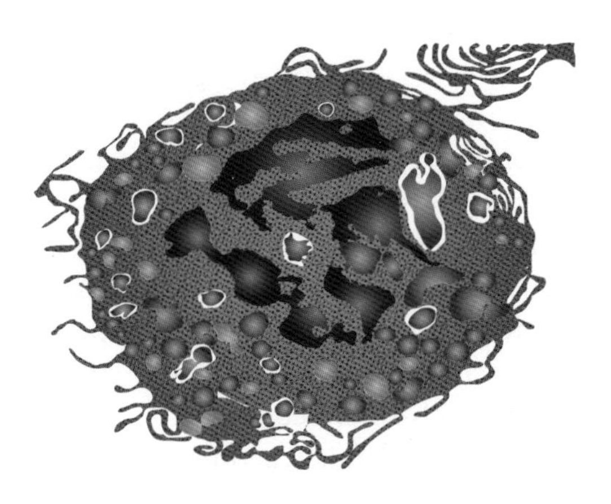

Fig. 6 Mast cell.

These cells are usually found in the structural compartment of the lymphoid organs such as the thymus, lymph nodes and spleen. However, they are also found in the bloodstream and other tissues of the body, such as the skin and the lungs. It is believed that they capture antigens or bring them to the lymphoid organs where an immune response is initiated. Unfortunately, one reason we know so little about dendritic cells is that they are extremely hard to isolate, which is often a prerequisite for the study of the functional qualities of specific cell types.

7. Mast Cells (Fig. 6) and Basophiles

The role of mast cells and basophiles in normal (healthy) immune responses is still very unclear, although it has been established that they can play an important protective role, being intimately involved in wound healing and defence against micro-organisms. Basophiles are mainly found in the blood, whereas mast cells are found in a large number of tissues. Mast cells are very close to basophiles. These similarities have led many to speculate that mast cells and basophiles are similar, but have "homed in" on tissues. However, current evidence suggests that they are generated by different precursor cells in the bone marrow. The basophile leaves the bone marrow when they are already mature, while the mast cell circulates in an immature form, only maturing once in a tissue site. Two types of mast cells are recognized, those from connective tissue and a distinct set of mucosal mast cells.

Both mast cells and basophiles are very much involved in the initial phase of allergic reactions, as both cells bear receptors of IgE antibodies on the membranes. Once the IgE-antigen complexes are bound to the membranes, the cells become activated, which results in the break down of the cell membrane and release of mediators. These mediators (such as histamine and prostaglandins) will then activate and recruit other cells, which will result in inflammation in different organs. Mast cells are mainly involved in rhinitis, asthma and urticaria, while basophiles seem to be more involved in severe generalized allergic reactions, such as anaphylaxis.

The Immune Response

1. Initial Phase. An immune response to a foreign antigen requires the presence of an antigen-presenting cell (APC) (usually either a macrophage or dendritic cell) in combination with a B cell or T cell. When an APC presents an antigen on its cell surface to a B cell, the B cell will start proliferating and producing antibodies that specifically bind to that antigen. Antibodies binding to antigens on bacteria or parasites will act as a signal for polymorphonuclear leukocytes or macrophages to start action, engulf (phagocytosis) and kill them. Another important function of antibodies is to initiate the "complement destruction cascade": When antibodies bind to cells or bacteria, a group of serum proteins called "complement" bind to the immobilized antibodies and help to destroy the bacteria by creating holes in them. Antibodies can also signal natural killer cells and macrophages to kill viral or bacterial-infected cells.

2. Phase Involving Lymphocytes. When the APC presents the antigen to T cells, the T cells will become activated. Activated T cells proliferate and start secreting different interleukins or cytokines in the case of $CD4^{+}$ T cells; in the case of $CD8^{+}$ T cells, they become activated to kill target cells that specifically express the antigen presented by the APC. The production of antibodies and the activity of $CD8^{+}$ killer T cells

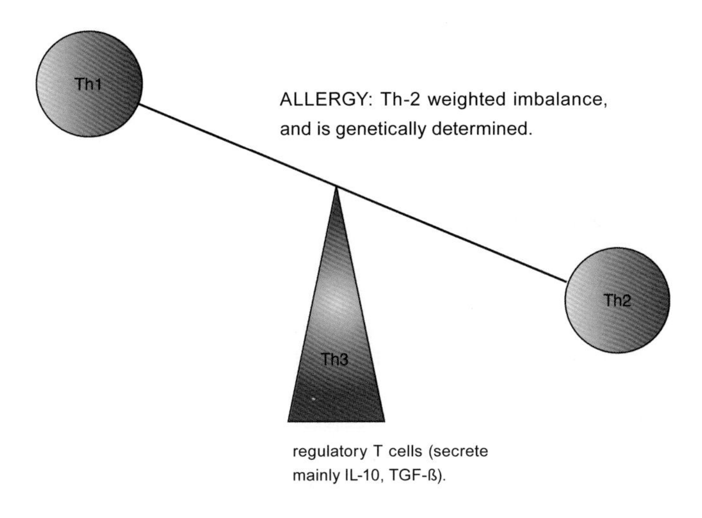

Fig. 7 The $CD4^+$ helper T cell subsets (Th-1 – Th-2 system + regulatory T cells). In allergy, there is an imbalance in which Th-2 features are dominant.

are highly regulated by **the $CD4^+$ helper T cell subset** (Fig. 7).

$CD4^+$ cells of subjects who are **genetically allergic** will start producing cytokines that will induce mainly an "allergic immune response." These $CD4^+$ helper cells are called T-helper 2 cells (Th-2), and one of the features of an allergic subject is that their T- cells have mainly a Th-2 profile (genetically determined) and that these cells produce cytokines that promote allergic immune responses. In contrast, the non-allergic type of T helper cells are called Th-1 cells. Another type of T helper cells (Treg cells), regulate immune responses, while yet another type, called Th-17 cells, is involved in inflammatory reactions, such as eczema.

An example of a Th-2-cytokine is interleukin 4 (IL-4) which stimulates the production of IgE. Other cytokines, called Th-2-cytokines, are IL-5 and IL-13. The ability of a person to secrete mainly Th-2 cytokines is genetically determined, leading to an allergic constitution, and putting the subject at risk for developing allergic diseases.

1. Common inhalant allergens
house dust mites, pollen
pets, moulds

2. Common food allergens
- egg, cow's milk, soy, wheat (children below 3-years old)
- peanuts, fish, shrimp (children above 3-years old)

Fig. 8 The most common allergens.

What causes allergy?

Usually, an allergic reaction is caused by a foreign protein that is harmless to a non-allergic person. This protein is called an "allergen." Almost any foreign protein can be an allergen to someone. The allergen could have been swallowed or inhaled. Sometimes the reaction occurs after contact of the protein with the skin or after injection of the protein into the blood by a bite (e.g. a hamster) or a sting of an insect. Some drugs which are not proteins can also induce an allergic reaction. This is because these drugs (such as penicillin) can bind to body proteins, creating a complex that can induce an allergic reaction. The drug is not a real allergen, and is called a "hapten" (= a small molecule that binds to own proteins, being transformed into all allergen).

Allergens (Fig. 8) are usually divided into two groups: **inhaled allergens** (house dust mites, pollen, cat or dog dander, etc.) and **food allergens** (milk, egg, peanut, fish, etc.). However, the distinction is not really strict as both types can induce reactions by either the inhaled or oral route.

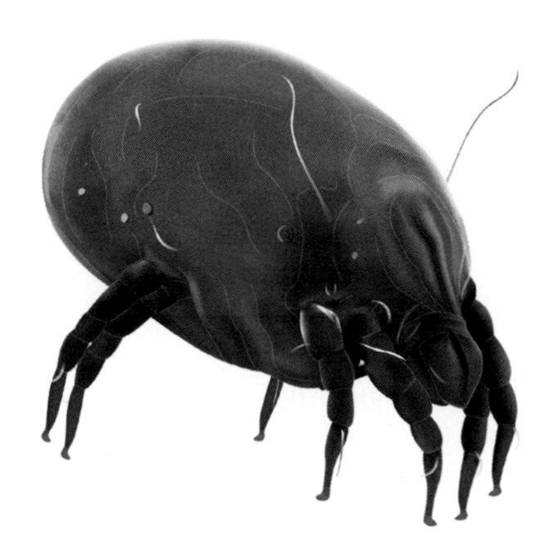

Fig. 9 House dust mite.

Inhaled allergens are further divided into indoor allergens (dust mites, cockroaches, animal dander) and outdoor allergens (different pollens from grasses, trees, and weeds).

Two examples:

- Dust from kitchens may contain food allergens that have become airborne during the cooking process. Ovalbumin, which is the allergen in eggs, can be found in sufficient amounts in dust to induce an allergic reaction through inhalation.
- Flour may contain house dust mites (especially from the group *Dermatophagoides farinae*). When ingested, these house dust mites (Fig. 9) are able to induce reactions that resemble food allergy (hives, swelling of lips and eyes) in a sensitive person.

The Mechanism of an Allergic Reaction

An allergic reaction is made up of **3 stages** (see Fig. 1): sensitization, mast cell activation, and prolonged immune activation (i.e. chronic inflammation). In the first stage, the body (immune system) encounters the foreign substance and identifies it as an invader. It then primes the immune system to recognize this invader as an enemy that needs to be destroyed in future encounters. However, instead of producing the right antibodies that might help to

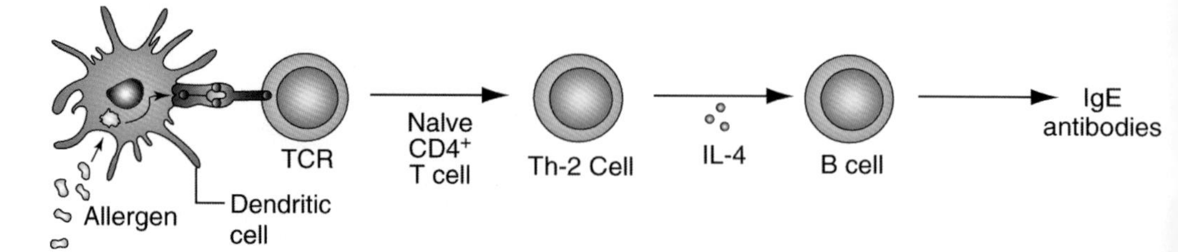

Fig. 10 Sensitization. Allergic sensitization starts with presentation of the allergen by a macrophage (or a dendritic cell) to a naïve (non-conditioned) T cell. When an allergic constitution is present genetically, conversion of the T cell into a Th2-cell takes place, thereby, inducing allergic reactions, including the production of IgE by B-cells.

destroy the invader, the immune system will produce IgE-type of antibodies that initiates allergic reactions.

Stage 1 Sensitization (Fig. 10)

The first time an allergen meets the immune system, no allergic reaction occurs. Instead, the immune system prepares itself for future encounters with the allergen. Scavenger cells called macrophages surround and break up the invading allergen. The macrophages then display the allergen fragments on their cell walls to specialized white blood cells, called T lymphocytes, which are the main orchestrators of the body's immune reaction. The T cells secrete interleukin-4, which activates B lymphocytes. These cells secrete IgE specific for that particular allergen. IgE will attach to cells of the immune system, namely mast cells and basophiles.

Stage 2 Mast Cell Activation (Fig. 11)

Stage 2, or mast cell activation, represents a later encounter between the allergen and the immune system and usually occurs within minutes after the second exposure to an allergen. IgE antibodies on mast cells, produced during the sensitization phase,

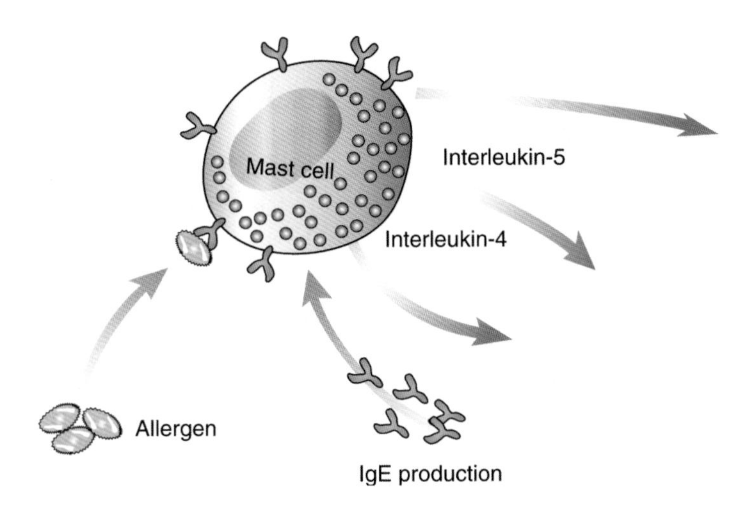

Fig. 11 Mast cell activation.

recognize the allergen and bind to it, forming complexes on the cell membrane. Once the allergen is bound to the IgE molecules, the membrane gets ruptured and the granules of the mast cells release their contents. These contents, or mediators, are substances such as histamine, platelet-activating factor, prostaglandins, and leukotrienes. Mediators are what actually trigger the allergy attack. Histamine stimulates mucus production and causes redness, swelling, and inflammation. Prostaglandins constrict airways and enlarge blood vessels.

Stage 3 Inflammatory Response (Fig. 12)

In Stage 3, tissue mast cells and neighboring cells produce chemical messengers that signal circulating basophiles, eosinophils, and other cells to migrate into that tissue, to help fight the foreign material. These recruited immune cells secrete chemicals of their own that sustain inflammation, cause tissue damage, and recruit yet more immune cells. This phase occurs several hours after exposure and can last for hours and even days.

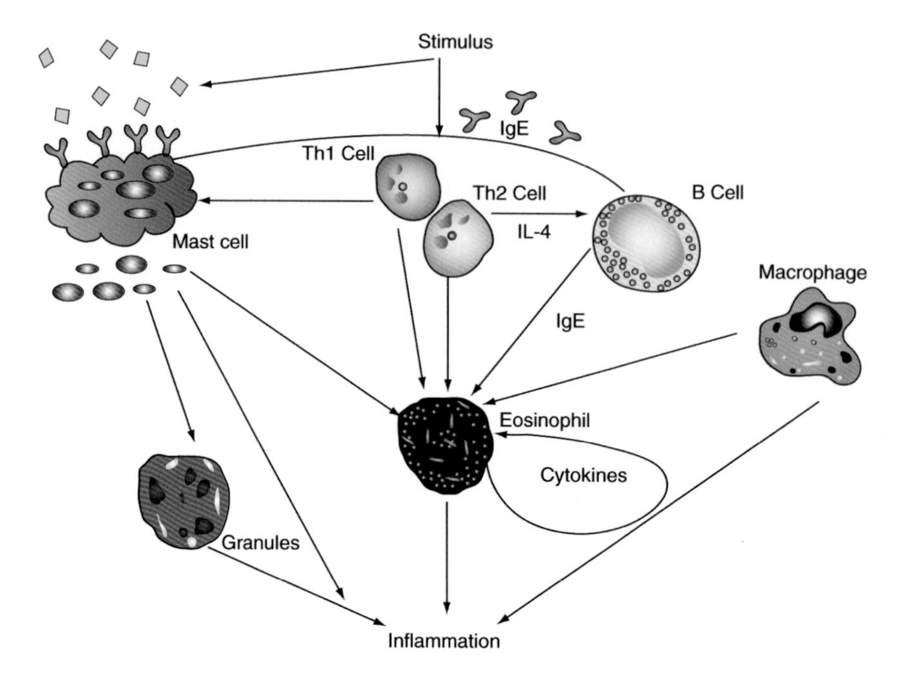

Fig. 12 Inflammatory response.

Parent's citations that are incorrect interpretations:

- My child is allergic to cigarette smoke
- My child is allergic to swimming pool water
- My child got allergy from the boy next door

1. Cigarette smoke, although very unhealthy, is not an allergen, but can cause all kind of irritative reactions to the airways. The same can be said of swimming pool water or strong perfumes, which can all irritate the airways (even in healthy persons).
2. Allergy is mainly determined by a genetic constitution and is not contagious.

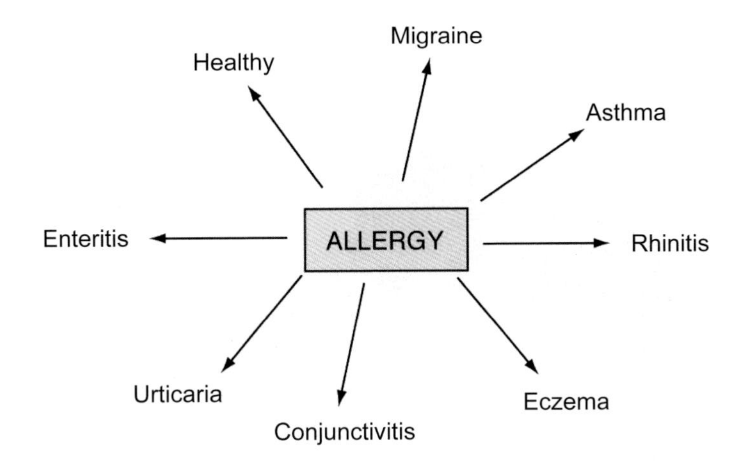

Fig. 13 "Allergy" and the different symptoms.

What are the main manifestations of allergy? (See Fig. 13)

Persons with a genetically determined allergic constitution are at risk to develop a number of diseases. At the moment, it is not understood why a certain allergic patient develops asthma, while another allergic person develops rhinitis or eczema. Researchers think it has something to do with local sensitivity of the "shock organ" or "end organ" to the allergy; however, it is also clear that all the symptoms of allergy can be caused by factors other than allergy, and can exist in themselves without allergy being involved. Therefore, for symptoms to develop, it has been suggested that more than just allergy is needed: there must be a specific local sensitivity of the end organ (lungs, nose, skin, etc.).

Allergy is also a very dynamic process, especially in young children: allergic diseases come and go in young children. In contrast, allergy is much less dynamic in adults, but rather a constant persistent disease, as adults do not tend to grow out of their symptoms.

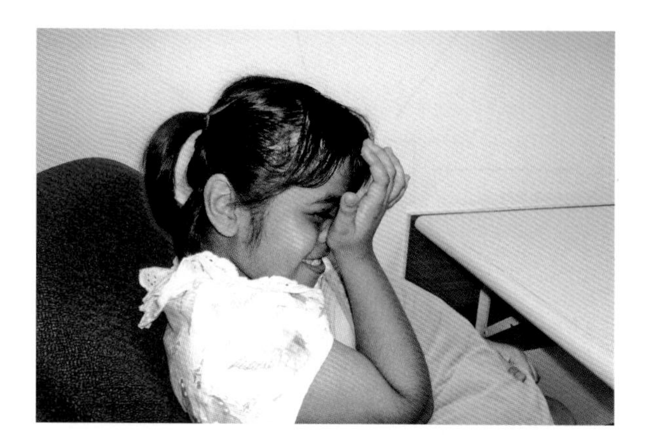

Fig. 14 Child with rhinits "allergic salute."

The three most common allergic diseases are: **rhinitis, asthma and eczema**, roughly affecting 1 in 4 children. Taking first place is rhinitis (allergy of the nose) which can be present in as much as 40% of certain populations (example: teenagers in Singapore). Second comes asthma (15 – 25%), and in the third place is eczema (15 – 20%), the latter especially in young children.

Allergic Rhinitis

Allergic rhinitis manifests itself as a blocked, runny, sneezing and itchy nose. The symptoms can affect the quality of sleep, learning, and social behavior. Allergic rhinitis can be chronic (perennial), or seasonal, and is than called "hay fever." It is an allergic irritation of the nose, where the inside of the nose becomes inflamed after being exposed to an allergic trigger. It is often associated with asthma, otitis media (inflammation of the middle ear) and sinusitis. Children who have allergic rhinitis may have dark circles under their eyes and they may use the palm of their hand to push the nose up in an attempt to relieve itching (which is known as the "allergic salute" (Fig. 14)).

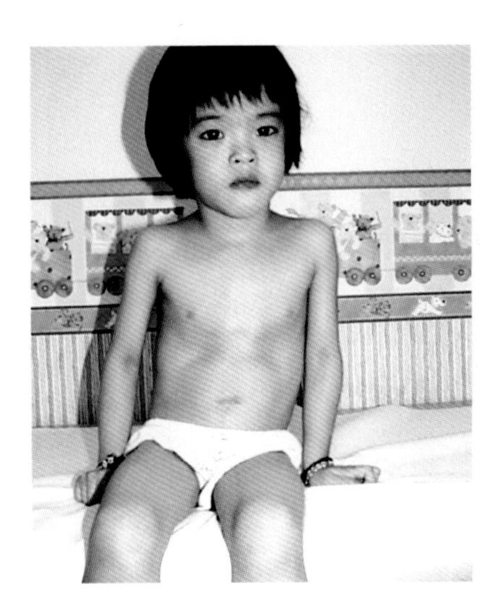

Fig. 15 Child with severe asthma. Severe attacks can lead to deformations of the chest. This girl presents with the so-called Harrison's sulci (caused by severe retractions of the ribs during acute attacks) (courtesy of Prof. Daniel Goh).

Asthma

The key symptoms of asthma are coughing, shortness of breath, wheezing and chest tightness. Asthma is an ongoing disease caused by inflammation of the airways, making it difficult to breathe. If the symptoms are severe and persistent, this can even lead to chest deformities (Fig. 15).

In young children, asthma is merely a non-allergic disease that is triggered by viral infections of the airways, often labeled as asthmatic bronchitis or wheezy bronchitis. However, the older the child gets the more allergy becomes involved, and from the age of 5 years, most children with asthma have an underlying allergy. In Singapore, the most common allergic trigger of asthma are the different house dust mites. Because both asthma and allergic rhinitis are diseases that affect the airways, controlling rhinitis will help control symptoms in people who also have asthma.

Atopic Dermatitis (Eczema)

Eczema mainly affects infants and young children, but, if severe, can

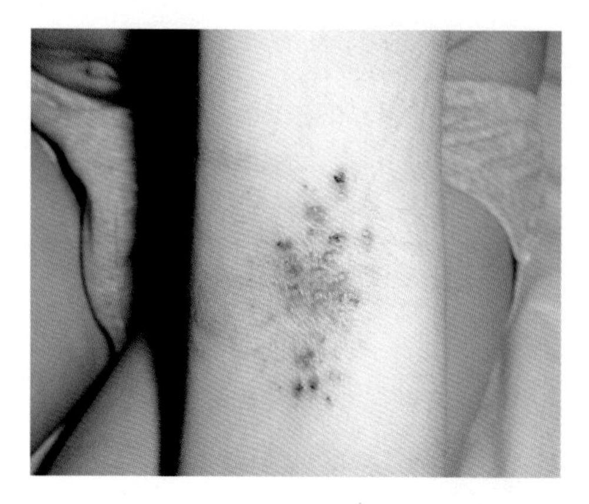

Fig. 16 Child with eczema. Elbow fold of a boy with chronic eczema: the skin is very dry and itchy. The lesions are infected as a consequence of scratching.

persist into adulthood. Eczema is often called "the itch that rashes." It is a red, inflamed rash most often seen on the arms, legs, ankles or necks of children. Because of the persistent itch, scratch lesions (open skin, crusts) that can become infected are often seen in these children (Fig. 16). Usually the itch gets worse in the early evening and at night, sometimes to the point of interrupting normal sleep patterns. Eczema has a strong impact on social life: children are embarrassed and feel isolated, leading to serious psychosocial problems. Eczema usually precedes the onset of allergic rhinitis and/or asthma. However, some children with atopic dermatitis do not develop respiratory allergies.

Related conditions to allergic diseases

There are several diseases that have an allergic component. If children have one condition, they are more likely to develop one or

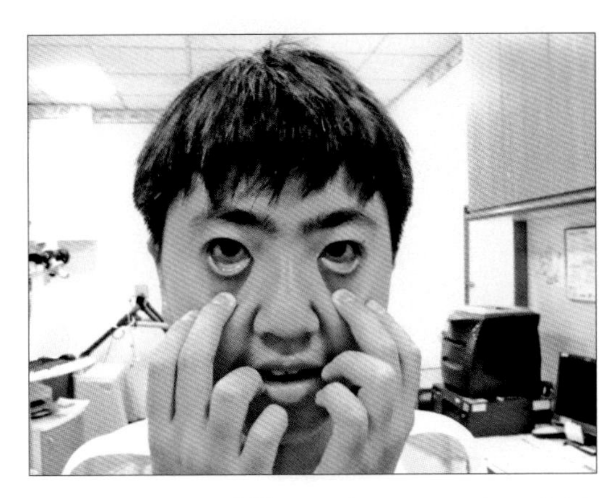

Fig. 17 12-year-old boy with severe conjunctivitis (red, itchy and swollen eyes) caused by an underlying house dust mite allergy.

more of these other conditions as well. Some of these conditions can be seen as consequences (complications) of an allergic disease, and appropriate treatment of the primary allergic disease will prevent these diseases from occurring.

1. Conditions related to Rhinitis

Conjunctivitis

Allergic conjunctivitis (eye allergy) can present as the only manifestation of allergy, but is often associated with allergic rhinitis, and is then called rhino-conjunctivitis. An inflammation of the whites of the eyes is the main sign of allergic conjunctivitis (Fig. 17). It is also indicated by redness, tearing, stinging, or pus discharging from the eyes. A solitary symptom of allergic conjunctivitis can be blinking, and children with the allergy are often referred to a neurologist because of a suspected nervous tic. Many children with allergic rhinitis develop the symptoms of allergic conjunctivitis and are sent home from school, even though allergic conjunctivitis is not contagious. In contrast, bacterial and viral forms of conjunctivitis are contagious, and are often preceded by an upper respiratory infection. Itchy eyes are the key distinguishing feature of allergic conjunctivitis.

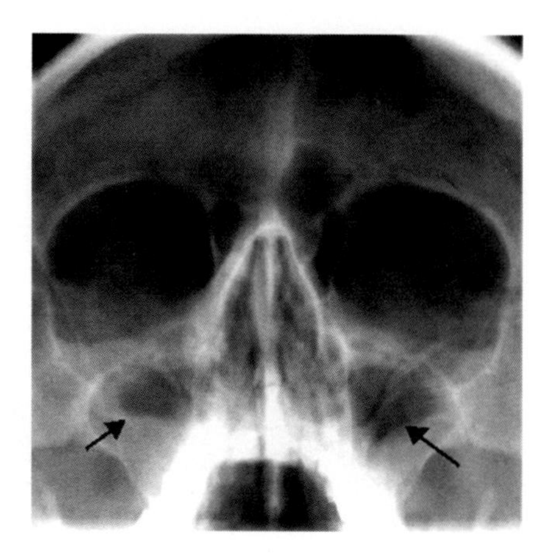

Fig. 18 X-ray of sinusitis. X-ray from a child with chronic sinusitis. Note the thickening of the mucosa in the maxillary sinuses. Thickening of mucosa is the signature of chronic sinusitis (while acute sinusitis presents merely as opacification of a sinus).

Otitis media

An inflammation of the middle ear, this is one of the most common childhood diseases that sends children to the doctor. It is also one of the most common conditions in young children for which antibiotics are prescribed. It can be ongoing, or can happen once in a while. Otitis media especially when recurrent, is often a complication of allergic rhinitis, especially in children under 3 years of age. However, otitis media can also be preceded by an upper respiratory viral infection. If not properly treated, over time, it can cause hearing loss and speech and language deficits. The earliest signs of acute otitis media are ear pain and discomfort. The child may be irritable and pull on the infected ear. Nonspecific signs associated with otitis media are fever, headache, apathy, vomiting, anorexia and diarrhea.

Sinusitis (Fig. 18)

Sinus involvement is a typical complication of allergic rhinitis, as most of the children with severe allergic rhinitis have an associated sinusitis. The combination is than called rhino-sinusitis. Coughing

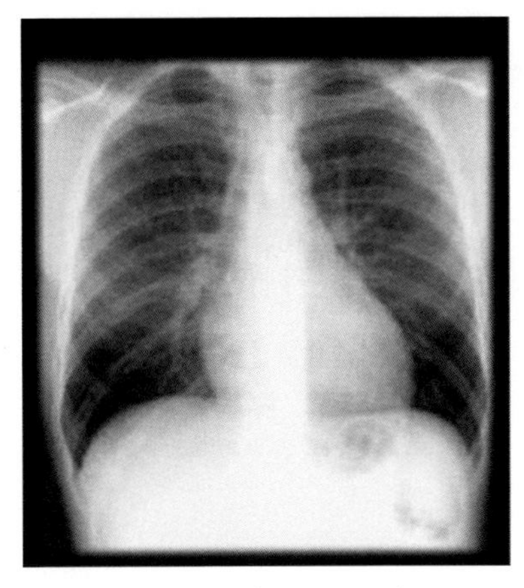

Fig. 19 X-ray of acute asthma. X-ray of a child with an acute asthma attack: the lungs are hyperinflated with air, because the air cannot get out of the lungs. On X-ray, this feature presents itself as "big, black, lungs" (mainly in the lower parts of the lungs).

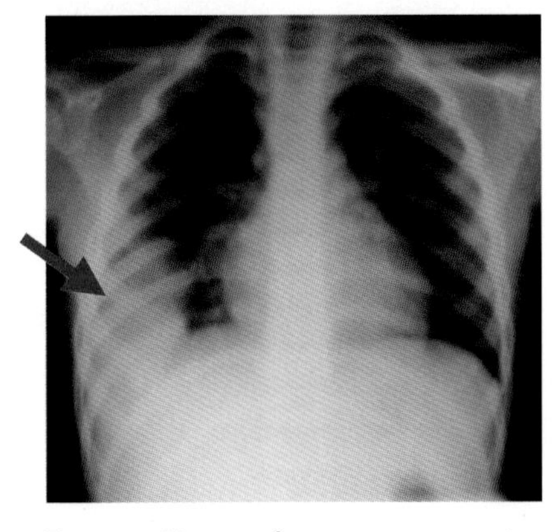

Fig. 20 X-ray of acute pneumonia. This might be a complication of untreated asthma. On the X-ray, the pneumonia is seen as a white spot in the right lung.

and dark yellow or green nasal discharge are the main symptoms of sinusitis in children. These children often have a so-called "throat cough," as a result of postnasal dripping. Another symptom of chronic sinusitis is recurrent infections of the throat (pharyngitis). Sinusitis and rhinitis can also occur with asthma, and more than 50% of individuals who have moderate to severe persistent asthma have chronic sinusitis.

2. Conditions related to Asthma

Infections of the lower airways

Untreated asthma may result in chronic hypersensitivity of the airways and to various infections (Figs. 19 and 20). Children with recurrent bronchitis or recurrent

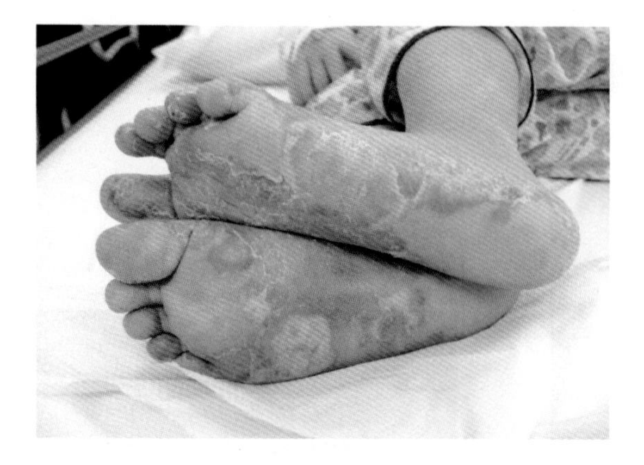

Fig. 21 Severe skin infection in eczema.

pneumonia often have asthma as an underlying disease. It is the rule that in children with recurrent airway infections, asthma should be considered in the first place. Other underlying conditions of the airways, such as a deficient immune system or structural abnormalities of the airways are far rarer than asthma.

3. Conditions related to Eczema

Skin infections

Various skin infections can occur in children with eczema, caused by viruses, bacteria, and fungi. Usually these infections manifest as exacerbations of the eczema (Fig. 21), but more typical lesions can appear, such as blisters, warts, and areas of pus formation. These infections need specific treatment, and appropriate treatment of the underlying eczema can prevent these infections.

Examples of skin infections in eczema are:

1. Different warts (including *Molluscum contagiosum*).
2. Bacterial infections: especially infections with *Staphylococcus aureus.*
3. Herpes virus infections, which can lead to *Eczema herpeticum.* This will be discussed further in the chapter on Eczema.

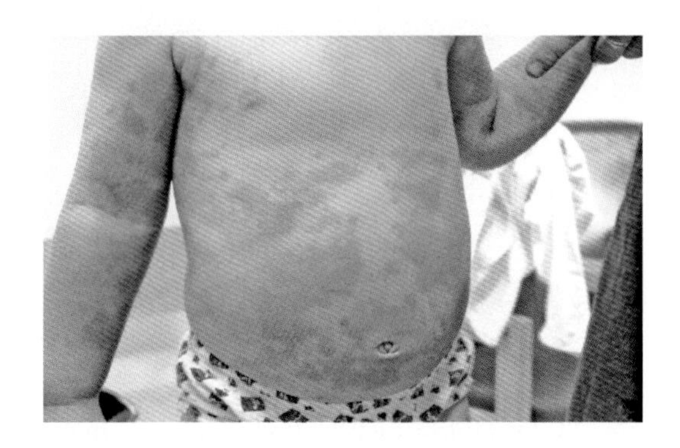

Fig. 22 Child with acute urticaria caused by an allergic reaction to antibiotics. The lesions are hived, irregular and very itchy.

Other allergic diseases

Allergy does not always manifest as symptoms. A large number of people are allergic without having symptoms, and they do not even know that they are allergic. Tests for detecting allergy in healthy children are positive in about 12% of them, and these children may not even experience symptoms of allergy.

1. Urticaria and Angio-oedema

Urticaria or hives can be divided into many types, such as acute urticaria (Fig. 22), chronic urticaria, and physical urticaria. Acute urticaria (or hives) can have a number of causes, including allergy, whereas the other types are less likely to be caused by allergic reactions. Urticaria is characterized by raised, irregular red skin welts (hives), made up of a combination of flare and wheal reactions that are very itchy, and that usually become worse after scratching. The rash can appear anywhere on the body, including the face, lips, tongue, throat, and ears. Welts may vary in size from about 5 mm (0.2 inches) in diameter to the size of a dinner plate, and they typically itch severely, sting, or burn, and often have a pale border. When urticaria develops around loose tissues, such as the tissues of the eyes or lips, the affected area may

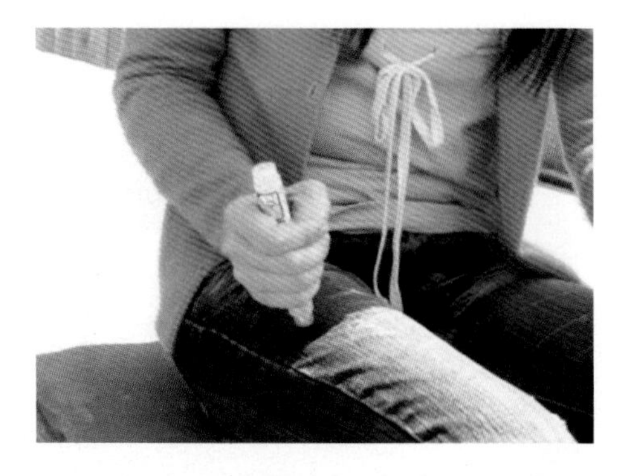

Fig. 23 Girl injecting herself with Epipen. In case of a severe allergic reaction, such as anaphylaxis (which can be induced by a food allergy), patients are instructed to inject themselves with adrenaline.

swell excessively. This is called angioedema (swelling) which is considered as a more severe manifestation than urticaria, but with similar etiology. Angioedema is considered as a vascular reaction, involving the deep dermis or subcutaneous or submucosal tissues, representing localized edema caused by dilatation and increased permeability of blood vessels, and characterized by the development of giant wheals. Angioedema can also occur in the throat, which can lead to swelling of the throat, and shortness of breath, which can be fatal.

The allergies that cause acute urticaria and/or angioedema are mainly allergies to various foods, such as peanuts, seafood, eggs, cow's milk, fish and others. A large number of drugs have been associated with urticaria and angioedema. One example is allergy to antibiotics (penicillin) which can cause severe urticaria, angioedema and eventually anaphylactic shock. Urticaria and angioedema can also be a consequence of an allergy to insect stings, for example, from wasps or bees.

2. Anaphylaxis and Anaphylactic Shock

Anaphylaxis is considered as severe generalized allergic reactions that involve the whole body. Usually its manifestations are urticaria, angioedema, severe rhinitis and symptoms of asthma. When it occurs with a drop in blood pressure (= shock) and decreased cerebral (brain) blood flow (unconsciousness), it is called anaphylactic shock (see Fig. 23).

Anaphylactic shock can lead to death in a matter of minutes if left untreated. Causes of anaphylaxis are multiple, and include foods, drugs, and insect bites.

In a substantial proportion of anaphylaxis, no cause is found despite all efforts, even in the most expert clinics. Doctors call such unexplained attacks "**idiopathic anaphylaxis**." The word "idiopathic" in practice means we do not know the cause. Worrying as it is, death from this is very rare indeed. However, there must be a cause or causes. However, the explanation is NOT psychological in the vast majority of cases. So in most cases this is a disease for which medical science has not yet discovered the cause. Some top experts who have studied hundreds of patients with idiopathic anaphylaxis believe that it is a disorder of mast cells, causing them to release, histamine and chemicals with similar actions spontaneously.

3. Gastroenteric Problems

Acute vomiting and/or diarrhea are seldom caused by an allergic reaction, except in infants, as a manifestation of food allergy, especially to cow's milk. Gastroenteric symptoms in older children are usually due to other causes, although allergic reactions to food causing these symptoms have been reported. In general, most of these gastrointestinal symptoms are caused by other mechanisms, such as infections, intolerance to certain foods (lactose, gluten) or after consumption of food that contains toxic substances.

4. Other Diseases in which Allergy can be Involved

A number of other conditions have been associated with allergic reactions, although the direct evidence for this is low, and although in most of the cases, allergy is not involved. Examples of this are: migraine, autism, behavioral disorders and kidney diseases.

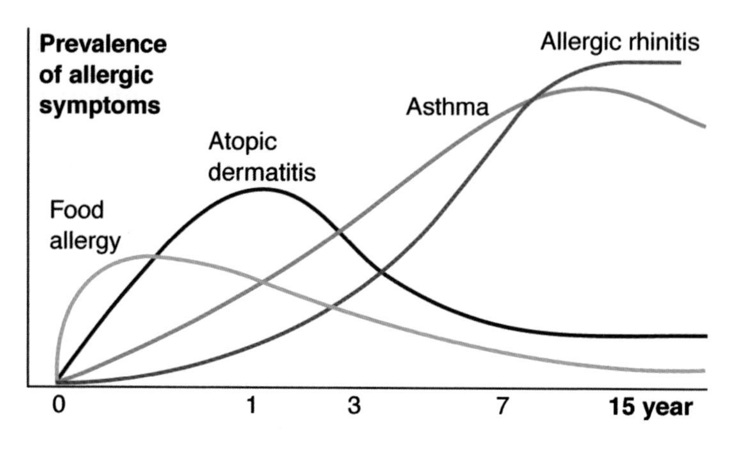

Fig. 24 The allergic march.

The Allergic March (Fig. 24)

In young children, eczema and chronic gastroenteritis are usually the first manifestations of allergy, while in older subjects, allergy manifests itself more often as a chronic or recurrent respiratory disease (asthma and/or allergic rhinitis). Furthermore, food allergy (egg, cow's milk) is the main type of reaction during the first year of life, while allergy to inhaled allergens (house dust mites, pets) seldom occurs during infancy (although sensitization could already have started). Children who are very allergic can develop different manifestations of allergy, according to age. Usually they start with developing food allergy (diarrhea, vomiting, failure to thrive), followed by eczema. These two events usually start during the first year of life. Subsequently, they will switch to other expressions of allergy, mainly the respiratory symptoms, such as allergic rhinitis and asthma. This phenomenon of switching from one expression of allergy to another is called the "Allergic

March." The exact mechanisms of switching from one expression of allergy to another are unknown. Probably, it has something to do with exposure to allergens and time for sensitization to allergens.

Conclusion

Allergic diseases are a result of allergic immune responses, which are largely genetically determined. They have a wide spectrum of manifestations, and can involve many organs. The most common manifestations result from allergic reactions in the skin (eczema and urticaria/angioedema) and the airways (rhinitis, asthma). However, other organs can be involved and it has also been shown that allergy can be found in completely healthy children.

2

Epidemiology of Allergic Diseases in Asia

What is epidemiology?

Epidemiology is the study of how often diseases occur in different groups of people, at the same time trying to answer the question why they occur. In other words, epidemiology is the study of the prevalence or incidence (see below) of diseases, its evolution with time (increasing or decreasing diseases) and its underlying risk factors. Therefore, epidemiological information is very useful (especially the identification of risk factors) for the planning and evaluation of strategies to prevent illnesses. Such information is also useful as a guide to the management of patients in whom the disease already developed.

Like the clinical findings, and the underlying mechanisms (pathophysiology), epidemiology of a disease or a group of diseases, such as allergic diseases, is an integral part of its basic description. Epidemiology has its special techniques of data collection and interpretation, and its necessary jargon of technical terms. Some examples of these technical terms are: population, cohort, cluster, endemic, pandemic, incidence, prevalence, etc.

In this chapter, an overview will be given of the current knowledge on the epidemiology of allergic diseases in children, especially in Southeast Asia.

Before that, some epidemiological terms need further explanation. These are:

1. **Population.** The group of subjects that is studied. This can be the general population or a more specific group, such as infants or children from allergic families.
2. **Prevalence.** The proportion of the population affected by a disease, at a particular time.
3. **Incidence.** The rate at which new cases of a disease arise in a population, also measured as attack rate.
4. **Morbidity.** Symptoms or illnesses produced by a certain disease in a population.
5. **Mortality.** Death rate caused by a disease in a population.

In most of the epidemiological studies on childhood allergies, **prevalence** is used as the preferential marker of the occurrence of an allergic disease.

An Example of the Use of Epidemiological Research

Studies performed in Germany during the 1970s and the early 1980s showed that the prevalence of allergic diseases was much higher in West Germany as compared with that in East Germany (children in East Germany more often suffered from respiratory infections). West Germany at that time was wealthier than East Germany, which was a communistic country, with a low standard of living, and with its many factories producing a high level of pollution. The fall of the Berlin Wall (Fig. 1) in 1989 offered a unique opportunity to compare the evolution of allergic diseases in the two populations, which are of similar genetic and geographic background, but which had been living under quite different environmental exposure conditions for over 40 years. In the former East Germany,

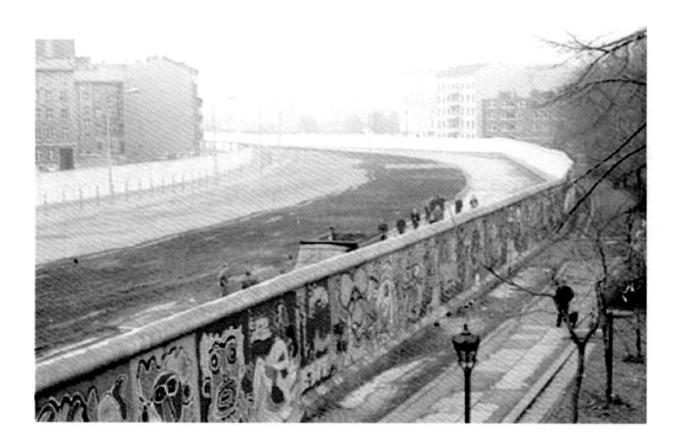

Fig. 1 The Berlin Wall. The fall of the Berlin Wall in 1989 offered epidemiologists a unique opportunity to study the evolution of the prevalence of allergic diseases, and the impact of Western civilization on disease occurrence.

tremendous changes towards a Western lifestyle occurred following the fall of the Berlin Wall. At the beginning of the 1990s, increased prevalences of allergic diseases were found in the former East Germany, resembling prevalences in the former West Germany. From these studies, it was concluded that a Western lifestyle is associated with the increased prevalence of allergic diseases. (Lancet (1998) **351**; 862–6.)

Epidemiology in allergic diseases: the hygiene hypothesis

The prevalence of childhood allergic diseases has increased over the past three decades, commencing from the beginning of the 1980s. The exact causes of this increase have not been identified, but it seems that a close relationship with *a "western life style,"* resulting in a decreased bacterial load (e.g. altered commensal flora) in young children, might be one of the main reasons for the increase. Some researchers call allergy: "*the prize you pay for luxury*," including being too clean and using a lot of medications, as it is likely that a decrease in stimulation of the immune system by bacterial contacts (i.e. bacterial load) can result in a higher risk for developing allergy. Although the evidence for this association is indirect (for ethical reasons, no controlled prospective studies have been performed on the role of bacteria in young children), a large number of observations point to that direction. The most important observations that have been made in that field, coming from different parts of the world, are:

1. Allergy is less common in large families, as siblings can produce an increase in contact with bacteria, infecting each other, thereby stimulating their immune systems. For the same reason, first born children are found to be more commonly allergic than their siblings.
2. Children attending day care centers early in life, and having contact with many other children, will develop fewer allergies than their counterparts who do not attend day care centers.
3. Contact with a pet (cat or dog) early in life seems to be protective for allergy. It is believed that this is due to contact with bacteria and their products (such as endotoxin) from the pet, stimulating the immune system of the young child.
4. Allergy is more common in clean families, where a lot of soap is used for washing the child many times daily.
5. Children living at big farms with a lot of cattle in Europe (Germany, Austria, and Switzerland) are less allergic than children living in cities.
6. Early use of probiotics (during pregnancy and the first six months of life) was found to have an inhibiting effect on the development of eczema, but no effect on respiratory allergies (asthma, rhinitis).
7. Early use of antibiotics, killing the bacteria of the child's intestine and upper airways, was found to be associated with an increased risk for developing subsequent allergy.
8. A similar observation was found for the early use of paracetamol, pointing to the fact that fever might have an inhibiting effect on the development of allergy.

Other factors that have been associated with the increased prevalence of allergic diseases are

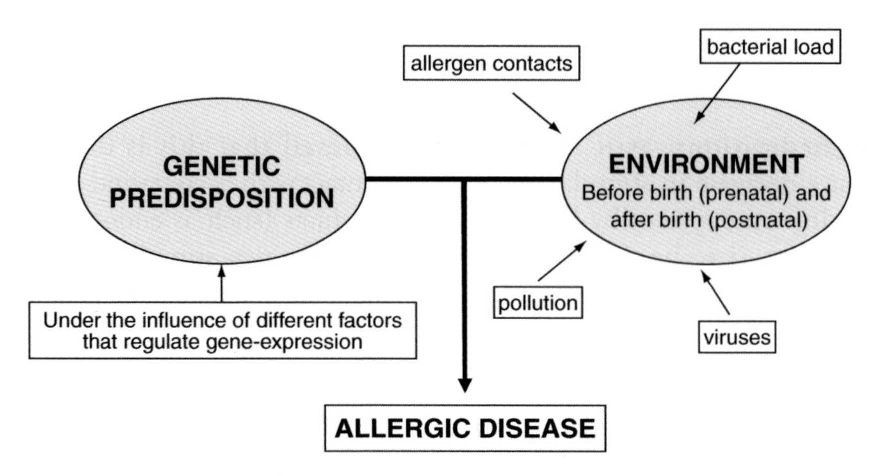

Fig. 2 Interaction of genetic constitution and environmental factors. Allergic diseases are the result of interactions of factors from the environment on a genetically predisposed person.

indoor and outdoor pollution, vaccination programs, and various viral infections (such as infections with respiratory syncytial virus) Obesity and an impaired physical condition have been found to be risk factors for asthma. However, it seems that these other factors are less important, and that ***a decreased bacterial load early in life*** is one of the main risk factors for allergy, in subjects with an underlying genetic constitution for allergy.

The cause of allergy is multifactorial, and the development of an allergic disease is the result of complex interactions between genetic and environmental factors (Fig. 2). Furthermore, it has now been accepted that allergic immune responses can start during fetal life. Nutritional, immunologic, and environmental factors acting during pregnancy all play a role in determining whether or not a child will be born with the propensity to develop allergic sensitization and subsequent allergic disease. Fetal exposure to different allergens has been demonstrated, including the presence in amniotic fluid of house dust mite allergens, and an active transplacental transport mechanism of different allergens (food allergens and inhalant allergens).

Epidemiology of asthma, rhinitis and eczema in Asia

A large number of national and international studies have been carried out, in most of the countries of Southeast Asia, on asthma, rhinitis and eczema. All these point to the same conclusions: asthma, rhinitis and eczema are the most common allergic diseases, and have increased during the last 30 years, although in most of these countries, there seems to be a plateau phase that has occurred from the beginning of the 2000s. One of the most important studies is the International Study of Asthma and Allergies in Children (ISAAC) (Table 1), which is a worldwide study that has been repeated almost every five years, starting from 1991, and that has provided data from most of the countries of the globe. Until the 1990s, most of the studies of the prevalence of allergic diseases had been undertaken in the UK, Australia, and New Zealand. The enormous participation in ISAAC Phase One, in which 700 000 children from 156 centers in 56 countries were included, demonstrated the worldwide concern about asthma and allergies. The ISAAC approach, using simple questionnaires, enabled the collection of comparable data from children throughout the world. The large variations in the worldwide prevalence of asthma, rhinitis, and eczema that were recorded, even in genetically similar groups, suggested that environmental factors underlie the variations.

Data from the ISAAC studies provided support for the hypotheses that economic development, dietary factors, climate, infections, and allergens might influence some of the variations in prevalence. ISAAC Phase Three, performed in 2002 and 2003, showed that in most Asian countries there was no further increase in the prevalence of asthma, as compared with that in the mid-1990s. However, prevalences of eczema and rhinitis still increased in most Asian countries.

Table 1 Prevalence (%) of Asthma, Eczema and Rhinitis in 2002 – 2003, in 6- to 7-year-old Children.

COUNTRY	ASTHMA	RHINITIS	ECZEMA
Hong Kong	9.4	17.7	4.6
Malaysia	5.8	4.8	12.6
Singapore	10.2	8.7	8.9
Thailand	11.9	10.4	16.7

Taken from the ISAAC Study Phase 3 (published in *Lancet* (2006) **368**: 733))

Most national studies, in which *rural areas* have been compared to urban areas, have shown that allergy is more common in rural areas. In a study from China, for example, it was found that asthma was more common in Hong Kong, as compared to mainland China (Beijing and Guangzhou). In the same study, it was found that allergic sensitization (as shown by a positive allergy skin prick test) in children was 41% in Hog Kong, while in Beijing it was 24% and in Guangzhou, 31% (Ref. *BMJ* (2004) **329**: 486).

Interpreting results of gross epidemiological studies has to be done with caution, as diagnostic criteria are usually based on questionnaire studies and not on clinical examination or diagnostic tests. Therefore, the results are very much dependent on how the disease was defined, and on the criteria that were used for making the diagnosis. In most studies, standardized definitions are used to detect the "obvious types" of asthma, eczema and rhinitis. However, we know that a lot of children have less typical symptoms or mild symptoms and, therefore these cases are not labeled as asthma, rhinitis or eczema. Furthermore, most studies are focused on specific age groups, and less data are available that cover all childhood ages. For instance, asthma seems to be more common in young children than in older children; but that type of asthma is usually non-allergic and these children tend to grow out of their asthma (see chapter on Asthma). The same can be said of eczema, this being merely a disease of children during the first three years of life. In young children, recurrent wheeze is a common symptom, affecting up to 30% of all youngsters. These children are usually not considered asthmatic, because the wheezing is merely a consequence of a viral respiratory infection. Most of these children are diagnosed as having "asthmatic bronchitis" or "spastic bronchitis." However, the underlying mechanisms of the disease are very similar to those of asthma (i.e. bronchial inflammation), and it has been suggested that these children be labeled asthmatic, this being a specific subtype of asthma: viral-induced asthma. Epidemiological data on viral-induced asthma are limited; however, from a number of studies, it was shown that this type of asthma has also increased in the recent years.

Studies in Singapore have found that wheezing had occurred in 23% of the children in their second year of life, while eczema was present in 22%, and allergic rhinitis (or rhino-conjunctivitis) in 8.4%.

In conclusion, since the early 1980s, prevalence data show an increase in asthma, rhinitis and eczema of about 0.5% a year. These diseases were prevalent in less than 10% of children in the early 1980s, while it is now close to 20% for asthma and eczema; in certain age groups (adolescents), prevalence of rhinitis has reached 30%. The exact reasons for the increase are still not known, but it is now generally accepted that a Western lifestyle, inducing a decreased bacterial load, is the main reason for the increase of allergic diseases.

Epidemiology of food allergy

The number of large epidemiological studies on food allergy is limited, and far more difficult to interpret, especially studies that used questionnaires to make the diagnosis of food allergy. This is due to the fact that food can induce a variety of symptoms that are not of allergic origin (intolerance, toxic, infectious, etc). Therefore, parents often believe that their child suffers from a food allergy, but specific testing on food allergy is negative, leading to a situation that food allergy is often over-diagnosed, not only by

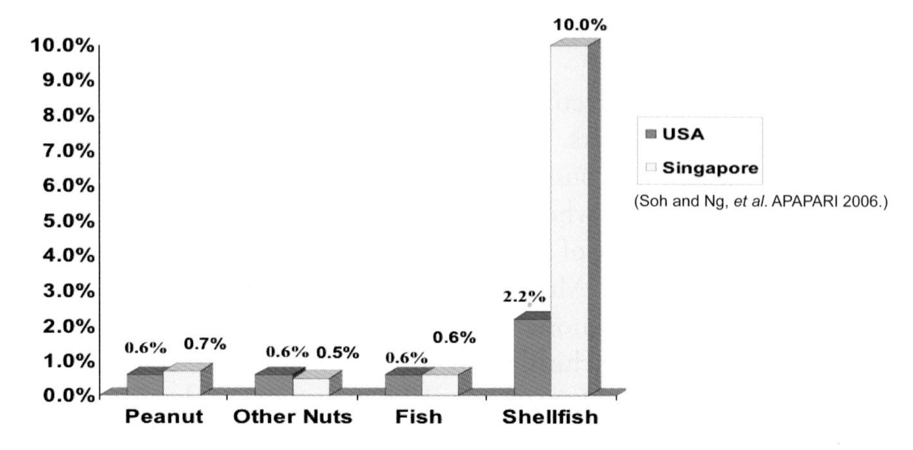

Fig. 3 Food allergy in Singapore teens. The study was carried out in 2005 in 24 schools, and involved 7697 students, aged 14–15 yr (Secondary 3). The figure gives a comparison with a similar study in the US, showing a higher prevalence in Singapore (courtesy of Prof. Lynette Sheck.)

parents, but also by physicians, especially when only relying on the history. However, from the studies that were performed it is now clear that food allergy is also increasing, especially in western populations.

These are the facts

1. In general, it has been shown that food allergies are less common than allergies to inhalant allergens, such as house dust mites. However, the prevalence of food allergies has also been increasing.
2. The prevalence of food allergy in the general population is around 2%, but higher prevalences have been noted in children, reaching values of 8%.
3. Studies in Singaporean children have found prevalences of food allergy of 4 – 5% (see Fig. 3). Similar prevalences have been found in China. In Korea (Seoul) and Japan the prevalence is higher, reaching 12%. However, the difference can be due to the methodology of the studies, and not reflecting a true difference.

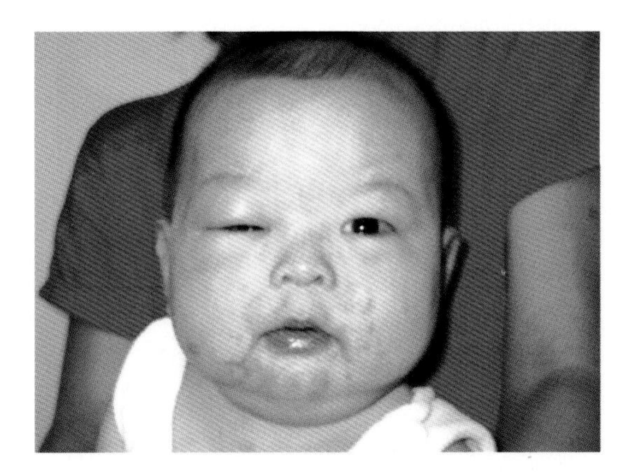

Fig. 4 Urticaria caused by a food allergy. Severe urticaria and swelling of eyes (angioedema) in an infant after drinking cow's milk (courtesy of Dr. Dawn Lim).

4. In specific groups of children with allergic diseases, the prevalence of food allergy is higher. In young children with severe eczema, for instance, the prevalence of food allergy reaches 90%. Prevalence of food allergy in asthmatic children is low, and is estimated to be lower than 5 - 10%.
5. About 2.5% of young infants (newborns) show an allergy to cow's milk protein (60% of these allergies are IgE-mediated).
6. Egg allergy occurs in 1.6% of young children.
7. About 0.5 to 1% of children show adverse reactions to food additives.

Asia is unique because of the presence of many different cultures and eating habits, which have resulted in the occurrence of unique types of food allergies (Fig. 4). However, little is known about the epidemiology of food allergies in Asia. The perception is that the prevalence in this region is low, but is likely **to increase** with the global increase in allergy. Unfortunately, data from many parts of Asia are still lacking. Large, well-designed epidemiological studies are needed so that the scale of the problem can be understood, public awareness can be increased and important food allergens in the region can be identified.

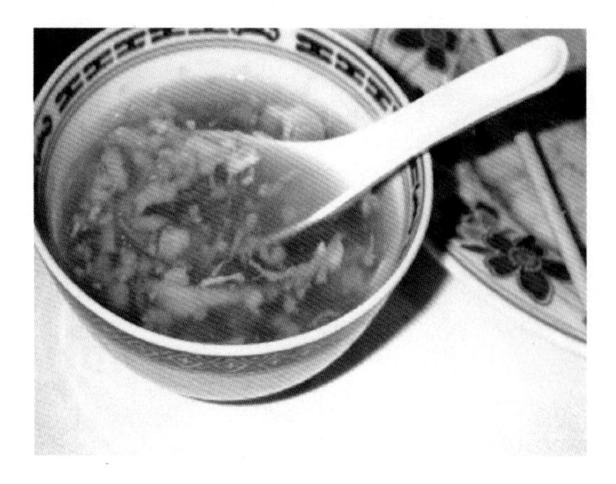

Fig. 5 Bird's nest, which is commonly given to Chinese children, and considered as "brain food" can induce severe allergic reactions.

Recent studies describing the pattern of anaphylaxis (i.e. severe allergic reactions to food) and the role of food triggers (Table 2) show that food is an important cause of severe allergic reactions in Asia. A study in Singapore showed that **bird's nest** (Fig. 5) **and seafood** are the most common causes of food-induced anaphylaxis. In contrast, peanut allergy (common in USA) and fish allergy (common in Europe) are uncommon in Asia. Other food allergies that have been described in Asia are allergies to buckwheat, chestnuts, chickpeas, and royal jelly. All these food allergies are rare, and epidemiological data on the subject are lacking.

Table 2 Foods Triggering Severe Allergy (Anaphylaxis) in Singaporean Children (1992–1996)

124 children with acute anaphylaxis at NUH		
		mean age (yrs)
1. Egg and milk	11 %	0.7
2. Bird's nest	**27** %	4.5
3. Chinese herbs	7 %	5.0
4. Crustacean seafood	24 %	11.0
5. Others *	30 %	7.0

* Chicken, duck, ham, fruits (banana, rambutan), cereals, gelatin and spices (Goh *et al.* (1999) *Allergy* **54**, 78–92.)

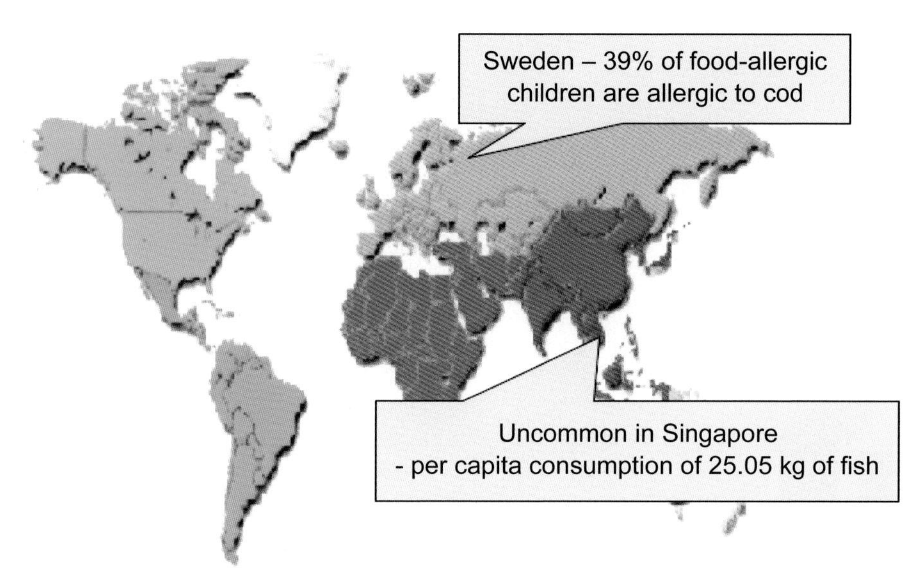

Fig. 6 Comparison of occurrence of fish allergy between Sweden and Singapore. Fish is an important element in the diet of the Singaporean population, with a per capita consumption of 25.05 kg. Singapore's local catch is not sufficient for the population and most of the fish available for local consumption are imported from the region. Singapore imports 241 000 tonnes of fish and fish products from the South China Sea every year. Despite this high consumption of fish in Singapore, the prevalence of fish allergy is extremely low in Singapore.

Conclusion

Epidemiological studies have shown that allergies have been increasing over the last 30 years. The exact reasons for the increase seem to be unknown, but are considered to be closely linked to a "Western lifestyle." The three most frequent allergic diseases are rhinitis, asthma and eczema. Allergy to inhaled allergens, such as house dust mites, is more common than food allergies. In Southeast Asia, a unique pattern of food allergy exists that is different from those in other parts of the world.

3

The Allergens

Allergic diseases are triggered by contact with allergens as it is the allergens that induce the allergic immune response in a genetically predisposed individual. IgE is the major immunoglobulin involved in the allergic immune response, leading to inflammation of shock organs, such as the nose (rhinitis), the lower airways (asthma), and the skin (eczema and urticaria). Without contact with allergens there would be no allergic reactions, and no allergic disease.

Therefore, it is useful to take a closer look at these allergens, which are completely harmless to non-allergic people, as everybody comes in contact with thousands of allergens, every day, by inhaling, touching, or ingesting.

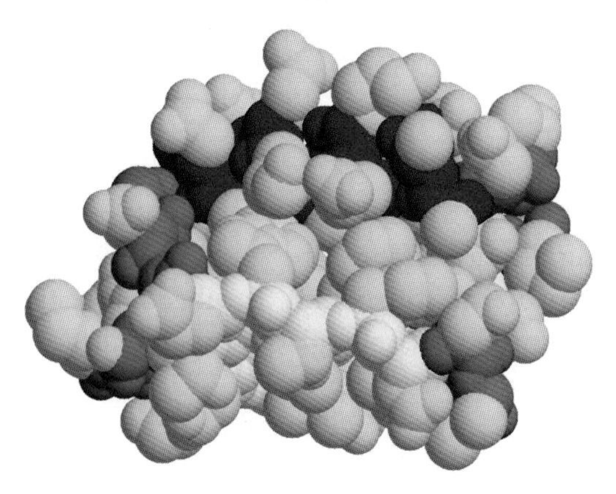

Fig. 1 Allergen (Protein). Proteins are large and complex molecules made of amino acids arranged in a linear chain. Like other biological macromolecules such as polysaccharides and nucleic acids, proteins are essential parts of organisms and participate in cell processes. Many proteins function as enzymes, and are vital to metabolism. Proteins also can have structural or mechanical functions, such as actin or myosin in muscle. Proteins are also necessary in animals' diets, since animals cannot synthesize all the amino acids they need and must obtain essential amino acids from food. Through the process of digestion, animals break down ingested protein into free amino acids that are then used in metabolism.

What are allergens?

Allergens are complex molecules that belong to the group of **proteins** (Fig. 1). Other complex molecules, such as sugars or lipids, are not allergens. Protein is often regarded as just something that we eat. It is, in fact, an organic compound containing hydrogen, oxygen, and nitrogen, which form an important part of living organisms.

Allergens are foreign proteins to which the body develops an allergic reaction. To non-allergic people, allergens are completely harmless. Therefore, an allergen is considered to be a substance capable of causing an allergic reaction because of an individual's sensitivity to that substance. There are two groups of allergens: **inhaled allergens and food allergens**. Furthermore, the inhaled allergens are divided in two groups: outdoor allergens (such as pollen) and indoor allergens (such as house dust mites). In this chapter, the most prevalent allergens will be discussed.

An exception on this is in the field of drug allergy. Drugs are usually not proteins, but small molecules that can induce allergic reactions by binding to the proteins of the body. Drugs that have the ability to bind to proteins are called **haptens**. A typical example is penicillin.

House dust mites (Fig. 2)

For a long time, it was observed that contact with dust could induce allergic reactions, such as asthma attacks. However, it was only in 1966 that Voorhorst and co-workers (The Netherlands) discovered it was the house dust mites in dust that were responsible for the allergic symptoms. House dust mites are found almost all over the world, especially in humid areas, and up to 30% of populations have been found to have positive allergy tests to at least one dust mite species. Sensitization to house dust mites is strongly associated with the three major allergic diseases: asthma, rhinitis, and atopic dermatitis. Evidence for the efficacy of avoidance of dust mites and their allergens in the treatment of these diseases comes from experiments in which patients' symptoms improved when they were removed from their houses and from successful controlled trials of avoidance in patients' houses. Allergens from house dust mites are the most prevalent type of indoor allergens. They can be found in mattresses, pillows, bedsheets, clothes, soft toys, sofas, and carpets. Even human hair can contain house dust mites.

There are many species of house dust mites (Fig. 3). However, allergic symptoms are mainly (but not exclusively) induced by **three species**: *Dermatophagoides pteronyssinus* and *Dermatophagoides farinae*, which are found worldwide, especially in temperate climates, but also in the tropics, and also a tropical mite (a storage mite) *Blomia tropicalis*, which is the most prevalent mite in the tropics, including Singapore.

Features of house dust mites:

- A house dust mite has a length of about 0.3 mm and can only be seen under a microscope.

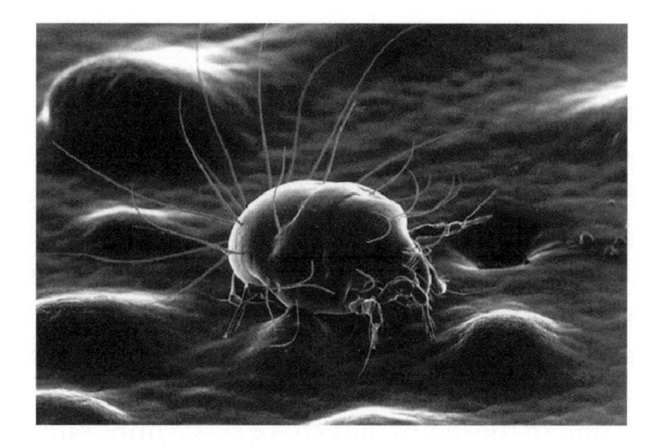

Fig. 2 House dust mite. Electron micrograph of *Blomia tropicalis*, the major tropical dust mite causing allergic symptoms in tropical regions.

Abbreviated classification of phylum Arthropoda

Phylum Arthropoda
- 1. Subphylum Uniramia
  - Class Insecta (insects)
  - Class Myriapoda (centipedes, millipedes)
- 2. Subphylum Crustacea
  - Class Malacostraca (crayfish, lobsters, crabs)
  - Class Maxillopoda (copepods)
- 3. Subphylum Chelicerata (Cheliceriformes)
  - Class Merostomata (horseshoe crabs)
  - Class Pycnogonida (sea spiders)
  - Class Arachnida
    - Order Aranea (spiders)
    - Order Opiliones (daddy longlegs)
    - Order Scorpiones
    - Order Pseudoscorpiones
    - Order Solifugae (whipscorpions)
    - Order Acari
      - Suborder Mesostigmata (free-living, predaceous, and parasitic mites)
      - Suborder Prostigmata (chiggers, follicle mites)
      - Suborder Metastigmata (ticks)
      - Suborder Astigmata (house dust, storage, & scabies mites)
      - Suborder Oribatids (soil mites)

The 3 mites that are mainly involved in allergy are:

1. *Dermatophagoides pteronyssinus* (Europe)
2. *Dermatophagoides farinae* (USA)
3. *Blomia tropicalis* (tropical regions)

Source: *J Allergy Clin Immunol* (2001) **107**: S406.

Fig. 3 Table of classication of mites. House dust mites are arthropods belonging to the subphylum chelicerata, class arachnida, order acari, and suborder astigmata. Other suborders of mites include mesostigmata, metastigmata (ticks), prostigmata, and oribatida.

- House dust mites live preferentially in hot and humid conditions. They feed themselves with human skin, and are therefore very prevalent in bedrooms: in mattresses and pillows.
- House dust mites are rarely found in the mountains above 1200 m, due to dry and cold climates.
- Concentrations of house dust mites are very high in tropical regions. Mite bodies and mite feces are the sources of many allergens (divided into specific groups on the basis of biochemical composition, sequence homology, and molecular weight). Some allergens are components of mite saliva that is left in the environment. After death, allergens from body fluids may be released as the body disintegrates.

How to avoid house dust mites?

The highest concentrations of house dust mites are found in rooms where people live in (house dust mites feed themselves with human skin), especially in bedrooms (including in hotel rooms, especially of old hotels). As we spend most of our indoor time in the bedroom, it is important to reduce the concentration of mites there. Complete avoidance is impossible. However, there are measures that can be instituted to decrease the concentrations of mites in rooms below the sensitizing levels.

Simple but effective measure to avoid house dust mites are:

1. Don't use old mattresses (Fig. 4) and old pillows. Sunning of mattresses and pillows can be useful.
2. Wash bedsheets and pillowcases in hot water (60°C), and change them weekly.
3. Avoid beddings such as pillows and comforters that are made of natural materials (such as feathers) and replace them with items made from synthetic fibers.
4. Remove stuffed toys and thick heavy curtains in the bedroom, as they can trap dust.
5. Damp dusting should be used to clean surfaces. Avoid feather dusters.

It is important to mention that house dust mites should only be avoided in cases of an existing house dust mite allergy (proven by positive allergy testing). It makes no sense to avoid house dust mites immediately after birth in an attempt to prevent house dust mite allergy (such as extra cleaning in the bedroom of a newborn baby). In some studies it was shown that this approach can actually increase the risk of developing a subsequent allergy to house dust mites.

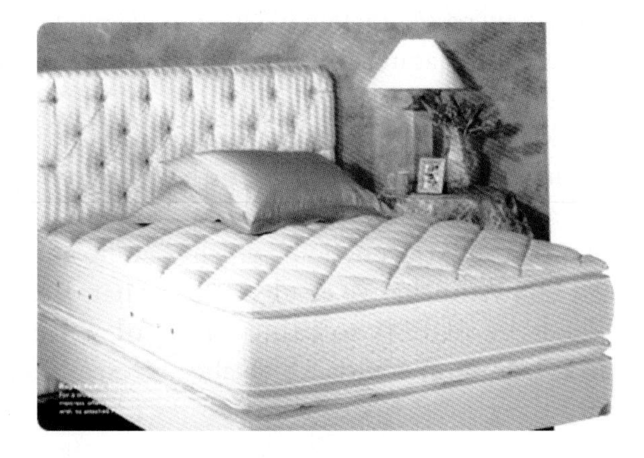

Fig. 4 Mattress. Old and thick mattresses and pillows are major sources of house dust mites. However, as house dust mites need our skin as their food, they will be found only in mattresses on which people sleep.

6. Air-conditioners, if used, should be cleaned regularly.
7. Avoid using carpets in bedrooms.
8. Sun mattresses and pillows.

Other measures that can be taken to reduce the levels of house dust mites are: covering pillows and mattresses with protectors; using a vacuum cleaner with a power brush - it is possible thus to reduce the number of house dust mites. It is important to note, when using a vacuum cleaner with water and filter inside, that the filter needs to be changed regularly to prevent growth of moulds and odour.

House dust mites as food allergens?

In rare circumstances, house dust mite can act as food allergens. This is illustrated by the story of a 14-year-old Chinese girl who was admitted to ER because of acute urticaria (hives) and swelling of lips and eyes (angioedema) after eating fried prawns. The girl was treated successfully, but we were left with a diagnostic dilemma, as the allergy testing (i.e. skin prick testing) to prawn were negative! Subsequently, the girl was also skin prick tested with a commercial extract of flour, which also showed negative results. We asked the parents to bring the flour from home with which the prawns were fried, and found that it had a brownish colour. The parents mentioned that the flour was quite old, having been kept for several months in the kitchen. Under the microscope we saw a lot of house dust mites in the flour, which were identified as being *Dermatophagoides farinae* (Fig. 5), a mite that likes to live in flour. Skin prick testing with the mite showed strongly positive results. Therefore, we could conclude that it was the ingestion of the mite allergens, living in the flour, that caused the acute symptoms of urticaria and angioedema, resembling an acute food allergy.

Cockroaches (Fig. 6)

Although there are no large epidemiological studies from Asia, allergy to cockroaches seems to be common, especially in combination with a house dust mite allergy, and is associated with

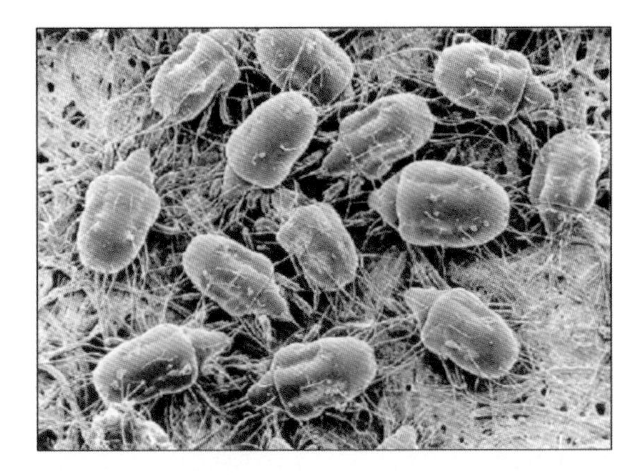

Fig. 5 *Dermatophagoides farinae* mites like to live in flour. Eating the flour can induce allergic reactions (urticaria) in people who are allergic to this mite.

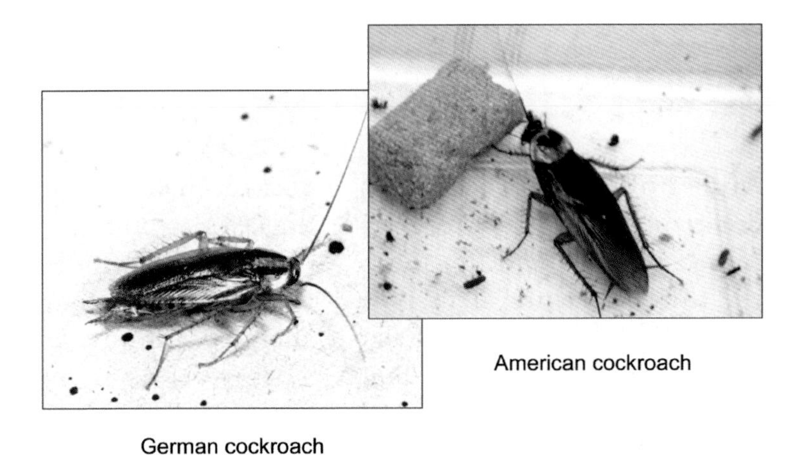

Fig. 6 The 2 types of cockroach.

asthma and rhinitis. Studies from different Asian countries, such as Korea, Hong Kong, Taiwan, Malaysia, Singapore, and Thailand have found that cockroach allergy is the second most important inhaled allergen (after house dust mites), producing allergic diseases, especially in low socioeconomic populations. An isolated cockroach allergy, however, is uncommon. Therefore, allergy to cockroaches is believed to be an expression of a severe house dust mite allergy. Both types of cockroaches, the American and German cockroach, can induce allergic reactions.

Symptoms of cockroach allergy can be: itchy rash (eczema), scratchy throat, or itchy eyes and nose. Some children develop severe asthma as a consequence of cockroach allergy.

Studies from the USA have shown that cockroach allergy is often associated with severe asthma attacks in inner-city children. In one study, it was found that 37% were allergic to cockroaches. In other studies, it was shown that 23% to 60% of urban residents with asthma were sensitive to cockroaches. Cockroach allergens are derived from the feces, saliva, and bodies of the insects. Cockroaches live all over the world, from tropical areas to the coldest spots on Earth. Studies have shown that 78% to 98% of urban houses have cockroaches, and the number of cockroaches per house can reach values of 300 000.

Pets: cats and dogs

After house dust mites and cockroaches, pet allergens (especially cats and dogs) are the third most prevalent type of inhaled allergens in Asia. In a study from Hong Kong, patients with allergic rhinitis showed the following prevalence of allergy: house dust mite (63%), cockroach (23%), cat (14%), dog (5%), pollen (4%), and mold (3%). Pet allergens can induce rhinitis, asthma, and skin allergies. Chronic exposure to a pet (every day) can result in a chronic state of hypersensitivity of the airways, such as chronic rhinitis and chronic asthma, and will make the airways more sensitive to other triggers such as pollution of viral infections of the airways. Therefore, a pet allergy can manifest itself as a recurrent bronchitis (asthma) or recurrent colds. The owner of the pet is usually not aware of the allergy (due to the chronic exposure), and it is only people who only occasionally come in contact with pets who will realize their allergy to the pet (due to acute exposure). Removal of the pet will then result in less sensitivity of the airways to other triggers. Washing the pet or keeping the pet outside of the house usually only results in a minor effect on the symptoms. Studies from the USA have shown that a large number of dust samples from houses or indoor public areas (such as schools or day-care centers) contain pet allergens, even dust from houses without pets. This is because cat and dog allergens can be carried on the clothing and hair of their owners.

Primary *versus* secondary prevention:

When a child is allergic to a pet, inducing symptoms that need treatment, it is advisable to remove the pet. The more contact with the pet, the more the symptoms can arise and the more severe the symptoms can become. This is called **secondary prevention**: meaning prevention of new symptoms in a patient who has already developed allergic reactions.

In contrast, **primary prevention** means prevention of symptoms in a child who is not allergic yet, but might be at risk to become allergic (example: a newborn from allergic parents). In a number of studies it has been shown that early contact with a pet (during the first months of life) might have a protective effect, preventing the development of subsequent allergy. There are two reasons for it: 1. Exposure to a high dose of allergen is able to induce tolerance (through specific IgG production) and not allergy (similar to what occurs after a vaccination or immunotherapy), and 2. Exposure to pets results also in exposure to higher concentrations of bacteria, which are carried by the pet. These bacteria are able to induce favorable immune responses.

Example: Studies from Europe (Switzerland, Austria, and Germany) have shown that children who live on a farm since

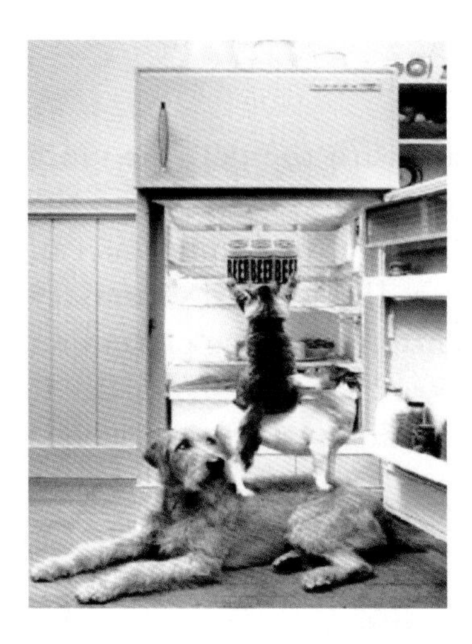

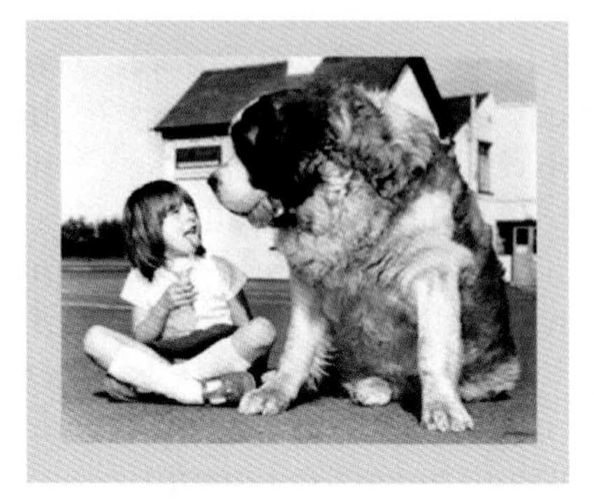

Fig. 7 Dogs and cats.

birth, and who come into close contact with cattle, will develop less allergic reactions later in life than children who are living in cities.

CAT

Cat allergy in humans is an allergic reaction to the major allergens from cats, which is a glycoprotein, called Fel d 1. This allergen is secreted by the cat's sebaceous glands, and it can be detected in the cat's skin and saliva. Studies from the USA have shown that allergy to cats is common. In symptomatic patients the prevalence can reach 25%. Cat allergy is more common than allergy to dog dander, which is related to the potency of cat hair and dander as an allergen as well as the fact that cats are not generally bathed. Cat allergen is produced in large amounts, particularly by male non-neutered cats, as the allergen is partially under hormonal control. The dander is very light and therefore constantly airborne (in contrast to dog allergen, which is a heavy allergen), sticky, and found in public places, even where there are no cats. This is due to the dander being carried on the clothing of people who have cats, then shed in public places. Therefore, cat allergen is a component of house dust, ***even in homes where a cat has never lived***. Moreover, the size of cat dander particles is extremely small and is inhaled deep into the lungs. Cat dander is therefore a common cause of allergic asthma, and cat owners who are allergic to cats are more prone to the development of asthma symptoms.

DOG

Dog allergy is less common than cat allergy, which may be related to the higher potency of cat dander as an allergen, as well as the fact that cats are not generally bathed at the same frequency as dogs. Regular bathing of pets, particularly dogs, could be expected to reduce much of the allergens released from the animal. The major dog allergen, called Can f 1, is primarily found in dog saliva, but also in dander (not in hair). Dog albumin, a protein found in the blood, is also an important allergen, and may cross-react with albumin from other mammals, including cats, mice, and rats. Dog allergen can also be found in houses without dogs and in public places. As with cats, chronic exposure to a dog can induce a permanent hyperreactivity of the airways, which can manifest itself as chronic or recurrent asthma and/or rhinitis.

HAMSTER

Allergy to hamsters (Fig. 8) is increasing, as hamsters have become increasingly popular household pets. It occurs especially in cities where people who live in small apartments choose to keep a hamster instead of a dog or cat (example: Tokyo). Hamster allergy can manifest itself as rhinitis, asthma, or eczema. The saliva of hamsters contains a potent allergen that is different from the allergens in dander. Therefore, hamster bites can result in severe generalized allergic reactions that manifest themselves as generalized urticaria and angioedema (swelling). Interestingly, the allergen in hamster saliva resembles house dust mite allergens. Children with an underlying allergy to house dust mites are at risk of developing severe reactions (even anaphylaxis) after hamster bites.

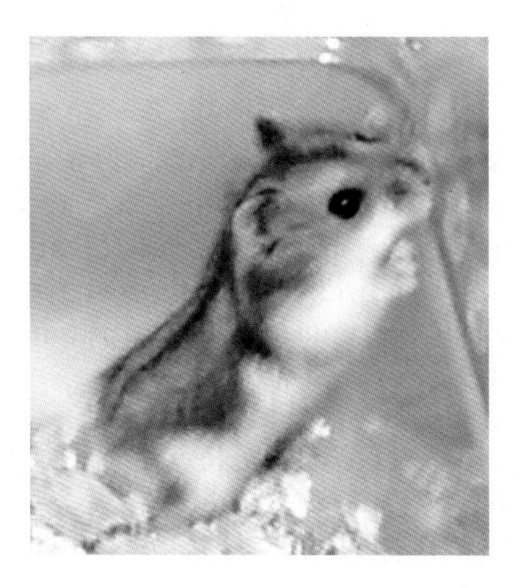

Fig. 8 Dwarf hamster. Hamster bites can result in severe generalized allergic reactions that manifest themselves as generalized urticaria and angioedema.

What is the best treatment for pet allergy?

The best treatment is to avoid contact with pets or their dander. Keep the pets out of the house, and avoid visiting people with pets. Avoiding cats and dogs may give enough relief, usually resulting in no further need of medication. Keeping the pet outdoors will help, but will not rid the house of pet allergens. Another option is to have pets that do not have fur or feathers. Fish, snakes, and turtles are some choices.

What if I want to keep my pet?

To test the effect of household pets on the quality of life, remove them from the home for at least two months and clean the home

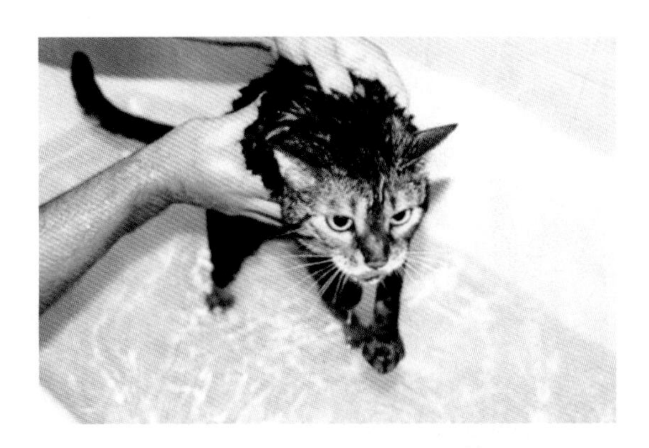

Fig. 9 Washing a cat decreases the risk of allergic reactions to the cat.

thoroughly every week. After two months, if the patient still wants pets, bring a pet into the house. Measure the change in symptoms, and then decide if the change in symptoms is worth keeping the pet.

If it is decided that the child wants to keep a pet, the pet should be barred from the bedroom. Keep the bedroom door closed and clean the bedroom aggressively:

- As animal allergens are sticky, the animal's favorite furniture should be removed, wall-to-wall carpeting removed, and the walls and woodwork scrubbed. Keep surfaces throughout the home clean and uncluttered. Bare floors and walls are best.
- If carpets are desired, select ones with a low pile and steam clean them frequently. Better yet, use throw rugs that can be washed in hot water.
- Wear a dust mask to vacuum. Vacuum cleaners stir up allergens that have settled on carpet and make allergies worse.
- Forced-air heating and air-conditioning can spread allergens through the house. Cover bedroom vents with dense filtering material like cheesecloth.
- Adding an air cleaner to central heating and air conditioning can help remove pet allergens from the air. The air cleaner should be used at least four hours per day. Another type of air cleaner that has an electrostatic filter will remove particles the size of animal allergens from the

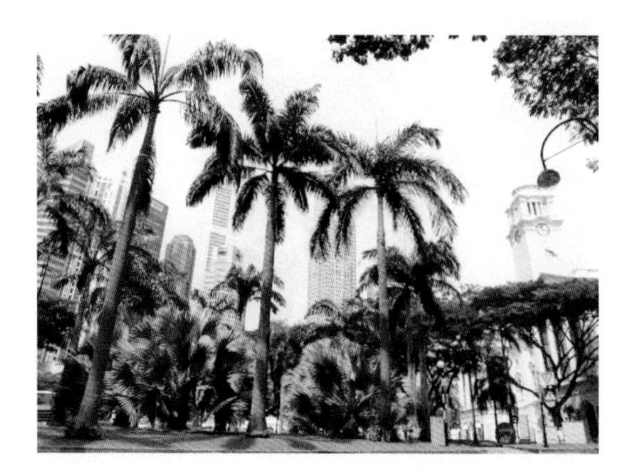

Fig. 10 Pollen in Singapore. In Singapore pollen allergy is rare, despite the fact that Singapore is a very green country and that a large number of different pollen can be found in the air.

air. No air cleaner or filter will remove allergens stuck to surfaces though.

- Washing the pet every week may reduce airborne allergens, but is of questionable value in reducing a person's symptoms.
- Have someone without a pet allergy brush the pet outside the house to remove dander as well as clean the litter box or cage.

Pollen

Pollen allergy causes important morbidity in areas of the world where there is a pollen season, which is usually in the spring. In tropical areas, such as Singapore, (without a pollen season) pollen allergy is rare, despite the fact that a lot of different pollen can be found in the air. It is however, the short and high peak of pollen concentration, occurring during the pollen season that is associated with allergic symptoms to pollen. These symptoms are usually

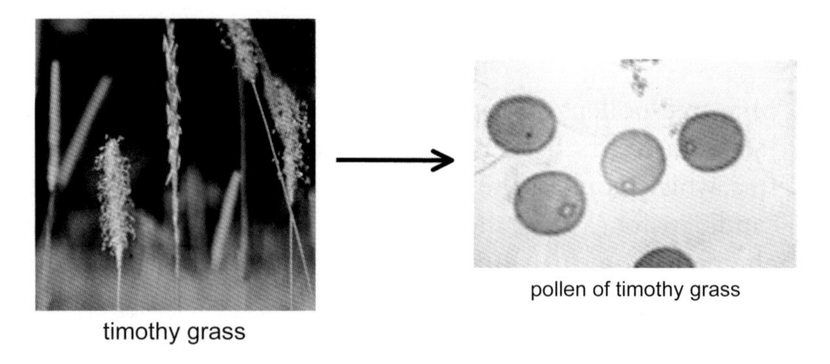

Fig. 11 Examples of pollen.

respiratory symptoms, such as seasonal rhinitis (also called "hay fever") and asthma, but symptoms of eczema and urticaria have been reported.

Pollen (Fig. 11) is a group of microscopic round or oval grains that are needed for plant reproduction. In some species, the plant uses the pollen from its own flowers to fertilize itself. Other types must be cross-pollinated; that is, in order for fertilization to take place and seeds to form, pollen must be transferred from the flower of one plant to that of another plant of the same species. Insects do this job for certain flowering plants, while other plants rely on wind transport. Types of pollen that most commonly induce allergic reactions are produced by the plain-looking plants (trees, grasses, and weeds) that do not have showy flowers. These plants manufacture small, light, dry pollen granules that are custom-made for wind transport.

Pollen of weeds, such as ragweed, has been collected 400 miles out at sea and two miles high in the air. As airborne pollen is carried for long distances, it does little good to rid an area of an offending plant, since pollen can drift in from many miles away. In addition, most allergenic pollen comes from plants that produce it in huge quantities. A single ragweed plant can generate a million grains of pollen per day.

The chemical makeup of pollen is the basic factor that determines whether it is likely to cause hay fever. For example, pine tree pollen is produced in large amounts by a common tree, which would make it a good candidate for causing allergy. The chemical composition of pine pollen, however, appears to make it less allergenic than other types. Because pine pollen is heavy, it tends to fall straight down and does not scatter. Therefore, it rarely reaches human noses.

Among North American plants, weeds are the most prolific producers of allergenic pollen. Ragweed is the major culprit, but others of importance are sagebrush, redroot pigweed, lamb's quarters, Russian thistle (tumbleweed), and English plantain.

Grasses and trees, too, are important sources of allergenic pollen. Although there are more than 1000 species of grass, only a few produce highly allergenic pollen. These include timothy grass, Kentucky bluegrass, Johnson grass, Bermuda grass, redtop grass, orchard grass, and sweet vernal grass. Trees that produce allergenic pollen include birch oak, ash, elm, hickory, pecan, box elder, and mountain cedar.

It is common to hear people say that they are allergic to colorful or scented flowers like roses. In fact, only florists, gardeners, and others who have prolonged, close contact with flowers are likely to become sensitized to pollen from these plants. Most people have little contact with the large, heavy, waxy pollen grains of many flowering plants because this type of pollen is not carried by wind but by insects such as butterflies and bees.

When do plants make pollen?

One of the most obvious features of pollen allergy is its seasonal nature (i.e. pollen season) (Fig. 12). Patients will only experience symptoms when the pollen grains to which they are allergic are in the air. Each plant has a pollinating period that is more or less the same from year to year. Exactly when a plant starts to pollinate seems to depend on the relative length of night and day, and therefore, on geographical location, rather than on the weather. On the other hand, weather conditions

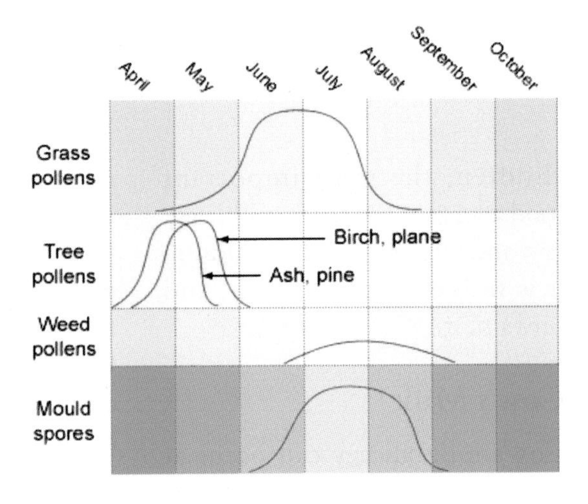

Fig. 12 The pollen season: an example of a pollen season in UK.

during pollination can affect the amount of pollen produced and distributed in a specific year.

A pollen count, which is familiar to many people from local weather reports, is a measure of how much pollen is in the air. This count represents the concentration of all the pollen in the air in a certain area at a specific time. It is expressed in grains of pollen per square meter of air collected over 24 hours. Pollen counts tend to be highest early in the morning on warm, dry, breezy days and lowest during chilly, wet periods. Although a pollen count is an approximate and fluctuating measure, it is useful as a general guide for when it is advisable to stay indoors and avoid contact with the pollen.

Important food allergens

Virtually all food can induce allergic reactions. However, most food allergies are rare, and there are only limited numbers of food that are frequently associated with allergic reactions. Compared to inhaled allergies (especially allergy to house dust mites) food allergies are rare (see Chapter 2 on epidemiology). In young children, the most important food allergens are cow's milk, egg, soy, and wheat. In older children, it is seafood, peanuts, fish, and bird's nest.

Cow's Milk

Cow's milk allergy can occur at any age, but it is more common among infants. Approximately 2% to 3% of infants have a milk allergy, and they typically outgrow it, before the age of one to two years. It is important to emphasize that allergy to cow's milk is not the same as **lactose intolerance**, which is the inability to digest the sugar lactose, which is rare in infants and more common among older children and adults.

Cow's milk allergy can develop in both breastfed and formula-fed children. However, breastfed children are usually less likely to develop food allergies of any sort. Occasionally though, breastfed children develop cow's milk allergy when they react to the slight amount of cow's milk protein that's passed along from their mother's diet into her breastmilk. In other cases, certain babies can become sensitized to the cow's milk protein in their mothers' breastmilk, but don't actually have an allergic reaction until they're later introduced to cow's milk themselves.

Cow's milk contains proteins, carbohydrates (such as sugars), fats, minerals, and vitamins. **Casein** is the principal protein in cow's milk, accounting for about 80% of the total milk proteins. The remaining 20% of cow's milk proteins are contained in the whey, the watery part that's left after the curd is removed. The proteins in milk are what cause allergic reactions in some people. A person may be allergic to proteins in either the casein or the whey parts of milk and sometimes even to both. The whey fraction contains mainly alpha-lactalbumin and beta-lactoglobulin and is most likely to induce allergy, through the production of IgE-antibodies. The whey proteins are altered by high heat, and so the whey sensitive person may be able to tolerate evaporated, boiled, or sterilized milk and milk powder.

EGG

Allergy to hen's egg is the most common food allergy in infants, especially in infants with eczema. An egg allergy can be found especially in infants with severe eczema. The exact reason for this

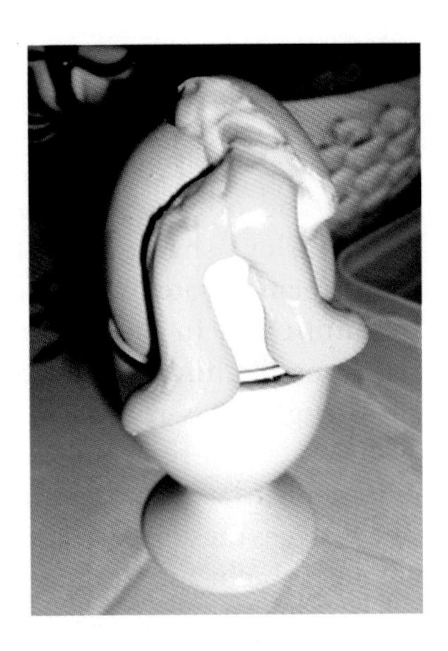

Fig. 13 Egg allergy is the most common food allergy in young children with eczema. The exact reasons for this are unknown, but it could be that this is induced by various contacts with eggs, early in life.

is unknown, but it is probably because eggs are widely used in many dishes. A second reason could be that egg allergens have been found to be airborne, and can be found in dust from kitchens. The major allergen of eggs is **ovalbumine**, which is present in large amounts in the egg white and much less in the egg yolk. Usually, children grow out of an egg allergy by the age of four to five years. If persistent in older children, egg allergens can induce urticaria and angioedema.

Vaccines and egg allergy:

Children with an egg allergy can be safely immunized. In the past, there was some concern about MMR vaccination (mumps, measles, rubella), but studies have shown that MMR vaccination is safe in children with egg allergy. The only exception is influenza vaccination, to which allergic reactions can occur in children with an underlying egg allergy.

WHEAT

Wheat and other cereal grains (rye, barley) share a number of allergens (proteins) that can be implicated in food allergic reactions in children, and that show high cross-reactivity. In addition, cross-reactivity with grass pollen has been reported. The allergens causing the reactions are the globulin and the glutenin fractions. Clinical reactions include eczema and urticaria.

Gluten (or gliadins), another protein, is responsible for celiac disease. It is important to note that wheat allergy and **celiac disease** are different conditions, and foods that are labeled as "gluten free" may not be suitable for people with a wheat allergy. When a person with celiac disease eats food containing the protein gluten (found in wheat and some other grains) it damages the lining of the small intestine, which stops the body from absorbing nutrients. This can lead to diarrhea, weight loss, and eventually malnutrition.

Patients who are allergic to wheat should avoid all food and products that are made from wheat and/or contain wheat in the ingredient list. This includes baked goods, baking mixes, breads, cakes, cookies, doughnuts, muffins, battered/fried foods, bread crumbs, cereals, crackers, croutons, creamed (thickened) soups, gravy mixes, and pasta.

SOY

Soy allergy affects approximately 1% of people in the United States. Soy, also called soya, is among the top eight most common foods that trigger allergies in children. In many cases soy allergy starts with a reaction to a soy-based infant formula. Although most children outgrow soy allergy by age three, soy allergy may persist and is becoming more common in adults.

In most cases, signs and symptoms of soy allergy are mild. Severe allergic reactions are more common with other food allergens than with soy, but in rare cases, soy allergy can cause a life-threatening allergic reaction (anaphylaxis). Deaths linked to soy allergy have occurred in people who also had both severe peanut allergy and asthma. You can reduce your risk of having an allergic reaction to soy by knowing as much as you can about soy allergy and how to avoid soy-containing products.

It is important to note that there is no cross-reactivity between FISH and SHELLFISH (SEAFOOD).

PEANUT

Peanuts and soybeans are ***two legumes*** (in contrast to tree nuts) that are responsible for a significant number of allergic reactions. In the USA, peanut allergy is the most common food allergy beyond the age of four years. In Asia, peanut allergy is less common, affecting less than 1% of children. Peanuts contain a number of allergens, traditionally classified as albumins (water-soluble) and globulins (saline-solution soluble). The latter is further subdivided into arachin and conarachin fractions. Peanut allergy can lead to severe reactions (anaphylactic shock), and fatalities from consuming peanuts have been reported, mainly in USA. Except avoidance, there is no treatment of peanut allergy. However, recent studies on immunotherapy to peanuts have been reported to show favorable results in adults.

Refined peanut oil was found to be safe in peanut allergic patients, whereas pressed (or extruded) oils retained some of their allergenicity.

TREE NUTS

Tree nut allergy is uncommon. In the USA it was found that tree nut allergy affects 0.6% of the population. Tree nuts that are most commonly implicated in tree nut allergy are: walnuts, cashews, almonds, pecan, pistachio, and hazelnuts. There is extensive cross-reactivity among tree nuts. Patients who are allergic to tree nuts do not necessarily need to avoid peanuts (a legume), and vice versa. However, in one study it was shown that about 35% to 50% of peanut allergic subjects are also allergic to at least one tree nut.

FISH

Fish allergy is less common in

Asia than in Europe or the USA, despite the fact that there is high fish consumption in Asia. Edible fish are predominantly found in the Osteichthyes, in which there are hundreds of species. Cod is the most common fish that can cause fish allergy. The major allergen of cod is Gad c1, which is a parvalbumin that has been isolated from the myogen fraction of the white meat. A similar protein, Sal s1, has been isolated from salmon. Unlike many other food allergens, the fish protein fractions responsible for clinical symptoms in some patients appear to be more susceptible to manipulation, such as heating or lyophilization. Furthermore, most patients allergic to fresh cooked salmon or tuna could ingest canned salmon or tuna without difficulty, indicating that preparation led to destruction of the major allergens. Nevertheless, allergic reactions following exposure to airborne fish allergens have been reported.

In Asia, it is mainly the tropical fish species that are consumpted, such as threadfin (*Polynemus indicus*), Indian anchovy (*Stolephorus indicus*), pomfret (*Pampus chinensis*), and tengirri (*Scomberomorus guttatus*). Studies have shown that these tropical fish are cross-reactive with each other as well as with Gad c 1 from Cod. Therefore, commercial tests for cod fish appear to be sufficient for the detection of tropical fish specific-IgE.

SHELLFISH (SEAFOOD)

Shellfish allergy is the most common food allergy in older children in Asian countries. A study on the prevalence of food allergy in older children in Singapore shows that about 10% of children report an allergy to seafood.

Seafood or shellfish consists of a wide variety of molluscs (snails, mussels, oysters, scallops, clams, squid, and octopus) and crustaceans (lobsters, crabs, prawns, and shrimp). The best studied allergens of this group are the shrimp allergens, of which **tropomyosins** seem to be the most important. Tropomyosins can also be detected in house dust mites and in cockroaches. Therefore, in Asia, a considerable number of children with a house dust mite allergy and/or cockroach allergy are also allergic to seafood, especially to shrimp. Furthermore, considerable cross-reactivity among crustaceans has been demonstrated.

BIRD'S NEST

In Singapore, bird's nest, which is considered a delicacy by Chinese people ("brain food"), has been found to induce severe allergic reactions, even anaphylactic shock. A study by the Department of Paediatrics at the National University of Singapore showed that bird's nest is the most common cause of anaphylaxis in children in Singapore, followed by crustacean seafood, egg, and cow's milk. Reactions to egg and milk occur mainly in infants while the remaining reactions occur in older children, with the oldest reacting to crustacean seafood. Similar reactions to bird's nest have been found in adults. The properties of the bird's nest allergens have been described. It seems that commercially available bird's nest from Sarawak (Malaysia) and Thailand are more allergenic than bird's nest from Indonesia.

Other allergens

Drugs

Virtually all drugs can induce an adverse drug reaction (ADR). The underlying mechanism of a large number of these reactions are unknown, and do not always involve IgE. The most common IgE-mediated allergic reactions to drugs in children are the allergic reactions to antibiotics, especially to the group of the beta-lactam antibiotics, such as penicillin or amoxicillin. In this type of reaction, the antibiotic binds to body proteins, acting as a hapten, transforming them to allergens. Other types of adverse drug reactions have also been described to antibiotics. However, it is the IgE-mediated reactions that are the most severe, leading to fatality. Other reactions are usually mild and reversible, although exceptions exist, such as the severe Steven-Johnson syndrome (Fig. 14) that can be induced by a large variety of drugs.

Data of population-based studies on ADRs, especially in large groups of non-selected children, are not available. In studies on hospitalized adult patients from the USA, the overall incidence of serious ADRs is estimated to be around 7%, with an incidence

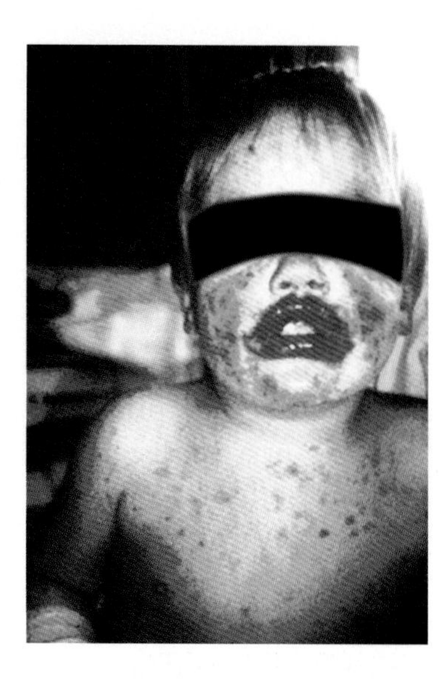

Fig. 14 Child with Steven-Johnson syndrome. Sometimes drugs can induce severe hypersensitivity reactions, such as the so-called Steven – Johnson Syndrome.

of 0.3% of fatal reactions. When both serious and non-serious ADRs are taken together, the percentage more than doubles, to 15% in hospitalized patients. In a retrospective study in children less than five years of age at the Children's Medical Institute, Department of Paediatrics at NUH, from 1997-2002, about 1% (0.7%) had a suspected ADR. Within this group, 30.3% were allergic to penicillin. A subgroup of these patients underwent allergy testing and it was found that only 13.3% of them had a true drug allergy. Drug allergy was more common in males and there were no cases of anaphylaxis to drugs described.

Biologic agents, such as heterologous antiserum, intravenous immunoglobulin (IVIG), and some vaccines, are complete proteins and do not need haptenation to induce drug allergy. Allergic reactions to these agents are common, and heterologous antisera are very potent allergens. Antisera in common clinical use are anti-thymocyte globulin and antisera to rabies, snake, and spider venom. Before using these materials, it is recommended to perform an allergy test (skin prick test). Skin test positive patients need to be desensitized. Anaphylactic reactions to IVIG are rare, but can occur in patients with a selective IgA-deficiency or in patients with common variable immunodeficiency who have anti-IgA antibodies developed prior to immunoglobulin infusions. In these patients, IVIG free of IgA should be used.

Latex

Natural rubber latex comes from a liquid in tropical rubber trees (*Hevea brasiliensis*). This liquid is processed to make many of the following rubber products used at home and at work: balloons, rubber toys, pacifiers and baby-bottle nipples, rubber bands, etc. In addition, many medical and dental supplies contain latex, including gloves, urinary catheters, dental dams and material used to fill root canals, as well as tourniquets and equipment for resuscitation. Non-latex substitutes can be found for all of these latex-containing items.

Latex allergy can be mild or severe, with symptoms such as: itchy, red, watery eyes, rhinitis, coughing and asthma, urticaria, and anaphylactic shock.

Who is at risk for latex allergy?

Health care workers and rubber industry workers seem to have the highest risk for latex allergy. Health care workers with hay fever have an especially high chance of developing a latex allergy, as 25% of all health care workers with allergic rhinitis show signs of being latex sensitized. People also at risk are those who have had many operations, especially in childhood, and people with spina bifida and urologic abnormalities.

As some proteins in rubber are similar to food proteins, some foods may cause an allergic reaction in people who are allergic to latex. The most common of these foods are banana, avocado, chestnut, kiwi fruit, and tomato. Although many other foods can cause an allergic reaction, avoiding all of them might cause nutrition problems. Therefore, it's

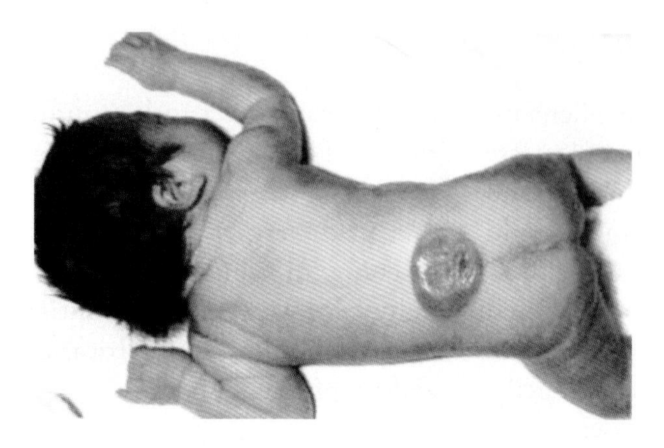

Fig. 15 Child with spina bifida. Latex allergy is on the rise in children with spina bifida. This indicates that the human race is getting more and more allergic, and that potentially everybody can develop allergic reactions, under specific conditions.

recommended to avoid only the foods that have already given you an allergic reaction.

The "latex story" in children with spina bifida.

The possibility of severe latex allergy in children with spina bifida was first raised in 1989. Since than research studies have shown that between 18% and 73% of children and adolescents with spina bifida are sensitive to latex as measured by history or blood tests. The type of allergic reaction experienced can range from watery and itchy eyes and/or sneezing and coughing, to hives (a blotchy, raised, itchy rash) to swelling of the trachea (windpipe) and even life-threatening changes in blood pressure and circulation (anaphylactic shock). Although the cause of rubber allergy in individuals with spina bifida (Fig. 15) is not known, it is theorized that sensitization may occur from early, intense, and constant exposure to rubber products through multiple surgeries, diagnostic tests and examinations, and also from bladder and bowel programs.

The "latex story" in children with spina bifida reveals that ***potentially everybody can become allergic***. The pivotal condition seems to be: early and repeated contact with an allergen, which will induce an allergic profile (Th2-profile).

4

Asthma in Children

Introduction

Asthma or bronchial asthma (BA) is a chronic disease of the lower airways or bronchi. Actually, BA is not one disease, but a group of diseases (different phenotypes), also called a syndrome: **THE ASTHMA SYNDROME**, of which the main feature is that the lower airways are very sensitive to a large number of environmental triggers, such as pollution (cigarette smoke, diesel exhaust particles), viral infections of the airways (such as common colds), and inhaled allergens (e.g. house dust mites, pollen, pets). Children with BA have overreacting airways, also called **airway hyperreactivity** or bronchial hyperreactivity. This overreaction of the airways causes an inflammation (e.g. red and swollen airways) with influx of different activated cells, swelling of the airways

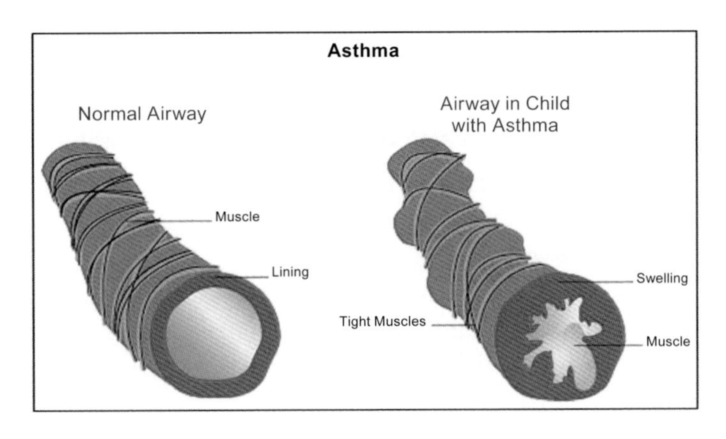

Fig. 1 Narrowed airways in asthma. In asthma the airways are swollen, leading to narrowing and difficult air passage.

(Fig. 1), constriction of the airways, and overproduction of mucus. The end result is that the airways are narrowed and hyper-inflamed, and if the triggering is constant (daily), this can result in scarring of lung tissue, and impaired lung growth or development. Asthma is therefore considered to be a condition of **chronic inflammation** of the airways induced and maintained by different environmental triggers, which differ from child to child. This inflammation and swelling reduces the amount of air that can pass through the airways, making breathing difficult and noisy (wheezing).

BA is increasingly common in Asia and around the world, especially among children, with a prevalence in about 20% of children. BA reduces a child's participation in activities and increases school absenteeism as well as parental loss in work days and anxiety. Allergies can often play an important role in childhood BA, especially in older children (over three-years-old). In contrast, in young children, BA is merely triggered by viral infections of the airways (common colds, flu, etc). These children show hypersensitivity to respiratory viruses, and allergy is only seldom involved in BA of young children. The viral-induced attacks of BA can be mild or very severe (sometimes needing treatment at the pediatric

1. Viral-induced asthma (mainly in young children)
2. Allergic asthma (mainly in older children, beyond 5 yrs)
3. Intrinsic asthma (caused by exercise, laughing, hyperventilation)
4. Secondary asthma (caused by other diseases, such as sinusitis, gastro-esophageal reflux, immune disorders, specific structural lung diseases)

Fig. 2 Types of asthma. The most common types of asthma. A lot of variations of this classification exist, and children can have an overlapping type. Moreover, in time children can switch from one type to another.

Intensive Care Unit). The good news is, however, that viral-induced asthma has a favorable prognosis, as most children will grow out of it by the age of six to seven. In contrast, if asthma is triggered by an allergy, there is a much higher risk that BA will persist into adulthood. Figure 2 shows the different types of BA in children. Different types can appear in one child, can overlap, and can alternate in time, as asthma is a very dynamic chronic disease.

Definition of bronchial asthma

A number of definitions of bronchial asthma (BA) have been circulating in the literature. It is important to note that BA is considered a **chronic disease** and that most researchers suggest a minimal duration of six months and/or a recurrence rate of at least three times before accepting the diagnosis. Sometimes in young children and infants, a duration of one to three months is proposed in which at least three attacks have occurred. Therefore, one or two episodes of wheezing are not considered as asthma yet, but rather as asthma-attack or viral bronchitis.

Definition of bronchial asthma

BA is than defined as a condition characterized by recurrent or chronic wheezing and/or coughing, with recognizable variable airway obstruction due to bronchial hyperreactivity, secondary to airway inflammation. It is important to recognize that asthma is a chronic disease, and that the airway inflammation is chronically present, even during symptom-free intervals.

Symptoms of asthma

Symptoms of BA can appear suddenly (attacks) or be present chronically (persistent). Symptoms include coughing (especially chronic cough and dry cough at night or after exercise), wheezing (best decribed as "a whistle on the chest"), shortness of breath, and tightness of the chest. Symptoms may differ from child to child. Usually, a child is labeled as asthmatic after having suffered from three attacks, or if the symptoms (such as a persistent cough) persist. In some children, coughing, especially at night, may be the only symptom of asthma, while in others, asthma may present itself as wheezing attacks or recurrent bronchitis, and even as recurrent lung infections (pneumonia). The most typical presentation of BA is the so-called "**asthma attack**" during which the child experiences sudden wheezing, coughing, and shortness of breath. These attacks can be mild or severe, and may need emergency treatment.

Non-typical presentations of asthma are:

- **chronic cough**
- **recurrent bronchitis (productive – asthmatic bronchitis)**
- **recurrent bronchiolitis (in infants)**
- **recurrent laryngitis – croup**
- **recurrent pneumonia**

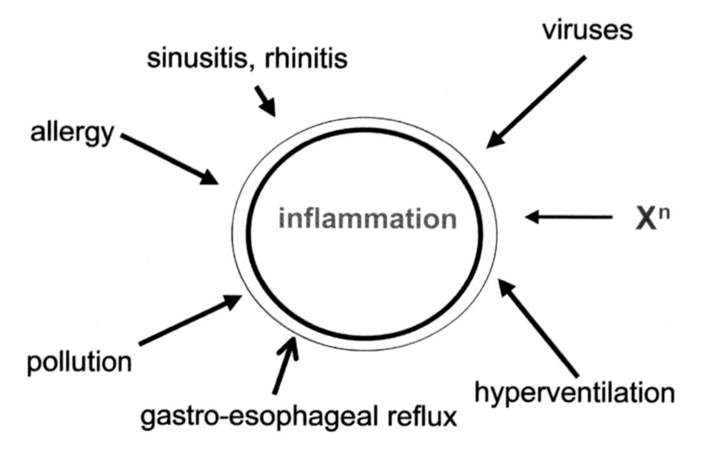

Fig. 3 An airway (cross-sectional) with the different triggers. Mechanisms of asthma: a large number of triggers can induce bronchial inflammation, leading to asthmatic symptoms. Some of these triggers have not yet been identified.

Determinants of childhood asthma

A large number of determinants factors have been identified, which can be divided into genetic factors and environmental factors.

Genetic factors

Studies in twins (monozygotic and dizygotic) suggest a genetic basis of BA, including BA without allergy. However, BA shows a large heterogeneity, and the manifestations of BA are strongly influenced by environmental factors. Accordingly, many children who develop BA do not have parents with asthma, and many parents with BA have children who do not develop BA.

Most studies on the prevalence of childhood BA have shown that the prevalence is higher in boys than in girls in the first 10 years of life. However, as children enter their teenage years, new-onset BA becomes more common in girls than boys, especially in those with obesity and early-onset puberty.

Environmental and lifestyle factors as determinants of BA (Fig. 3)

ALLERGENS

Especially in older children, allergic

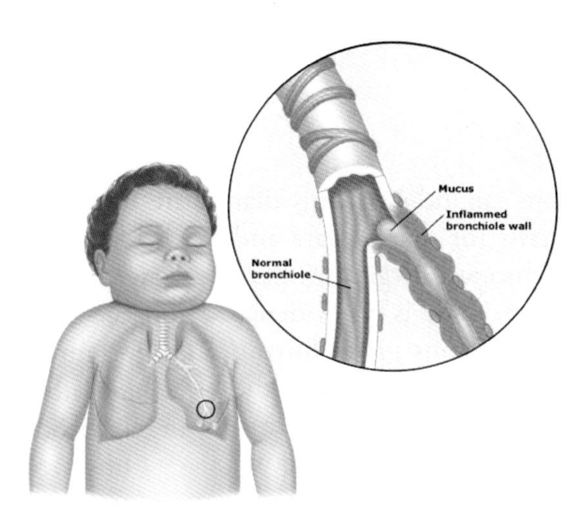

Fig. 4 Infant with bronchiolitis. Bronchiolitis in infants can be considered as a severe viral-induced asthma attack. These infants have fever, shortness of breath, and hyperinflated lungs, and need to be admitted to a hospital. A number of them will continue to suffer from recurrent asthma attacks.

reactions in the lower airways are important maintenance factors of BA. Exposure to allergens, especially to indoor allergens, is therefore considered a significant risk factor for allergic BA. However, clinical expression of the disease is variable, and depends on factors like the characteristics of the allergen, such as regional specificity, and indoor or outdoor presence. In infancy, food allergy with manifestations in the skin (eczema), the gastrointestinal tract or respiratory tract is more common than inhalant allergy. The presence of food allergy in infancy is also a risk factor for the subsequent development of BA beyond the age of four years.

INFECTIONS

Viral infections of the airways are the single most frequent trigger of BA symptoms in children. Some viruses can also exacerbate allergic asthma. Many viruses can trigger asthma, but human **rhinoviruses** are responsible for the majority of asthma exacerbations at all ages in children. In young children, however, **respiratory syncytial virus (RSV)** is one of the most common causes, leading to severe exacerbations, also labeled as "bronchiolitis" (Fig. 4). Furthermore, severe RSV infections can induce allergy that can persist for many years and lead to chronic allergic asthma.

To date, there is no evidence that vaccinations given during the first years of life increase the risk for BA or allergy. Exposure to antibiotics early in life (affecting the normal commensal bacterial flora of the intestines) has been associated with an increased risk for allergy and BA. Therefore, it is now recommended that antibiotics should only be prescribed in cases of suspected (or proven) bacterial infection, and not for viral infections, such as common colds.

TOBACCO SMOKE

Passive exposure to tobacco smoke is one of the strongest risk factors for developing BA symptoms at any age during childhood. In addition, maternal smoking during pregnancy results in impaired lung growth in the developing fetus, which may be associated with respiratory symptoms, including BA, in early life. In existing BA, smoking is associated with persistence of symptoms and may impair the response to asthma treatment. Although tobacco smoke is harmful to everyone, its detrimental effects are relatively greater in younger children due to their smaller airways. Therefore, avoiding tobacco smoke is one of the most important factors in preventing BA and other respiratory diseases in children.

Other irritants that can induce symptoms of BA are perfume and chlorine. Therefore, chlorinated water can be an irritant, especially from indoor swimming pools. A good ventilation system, however, can prevent this.

POLLUTANTS

The effect of air pollution caused by traffic or industry on pediatric BA has been extensively studied. In addition to their direct toxicity on the lungs, pollutants induce airway inflammation and may cause BA in those children who are genetically susceptible. Although pollutants are typically considered to be an outdoor phenomenon, high concentrations of pollutants can also be found indoors.

NUTRITION

There is no question that breast feeding is the best for all children, protecting them also from the development of allergic diseases, particularly in those with allergic heredity. Moreover, several studies have suggested that dietary factors, such as sodium content, lipid balance, and level of antioxidants, may also be associated with BA. These studies, however, have been difficult to control, due to the complexity of diet. Other studies have demonstrated that supplementation with omega-3-polyunsaturated fatty acids may reduce BA, but at the moment results have not been confirmed, and therefore, this regime should not be advocated.

EXERCISE

Exercise will trigger BA symptoms in the majority of children with asthma, and exercise-induced BA can also be a unique type of BA. Regular aerobic exercise, however, is crucial to healthy development, and should **not be avoided**. In addition, it has been shown that low physical fitness in childhood is associated with persistence of BA in adulthood.

STRESS

Psychological factors, especially chronic stress, can also affect the activity of BA. Furthermore, studies have shown that BA in children can also be affected by parental stress levels. Stress can exacerbate BA and there is a correlation between BA and psychological disturbances. Training in stress management may be beneficial.

Table 1 Common Triggers of Asthma, according to Age Group

	Infant	Preschool	Older Child
1. Viral airway infections	++++	+++	+++
2. Allergy	-	+++	++++
3. Pollution	+++	+++	+++
4. UAP	++	++++	++
5. GER	+	-	-

Legend: - = uncommon
+ = rare
+++ = common
++++ = very common

UAP = upper airway pathology (rhinitis, sinusitis, rhino-sinusitis)

GER = gastro-esophageal reflux

A true story

A 10-year-old girl with allergic BA knew she was very allergic to cats and that contact with cats could induce severe symptoms of BA. Her doctor told her to avoid any contact with cats as much as possible. One night, she was watching television. Suddenly, a cat appeared on the screen and the girl developed an acute attack of BA, although there was no direct contact with cats. The cause of the symptoms was stress, causing hyperventilation and symptoms of BA.

Asthma can appear at any age. However, the trigger factors can vary according to age: in young children (under the age of three), asthma is usually induced by viral infections of the airways (colds) and not by allergic reactions. In older children, allergy becomes increasingly more important, especially allergy to house dust mites, and also allergy to pets, cockroaches, and pollen. Food is very seldom a trigger of asthma, and if so, the child usually has concomitant symptoms, such as urticaria (hives) or swelling of the face (angioedema). Other triggers of asthma are: hyperventilation (exercise, laughing, and stress), diseases of the upper airways (sinusitis, rhino-sinusitis), pollution, and gastro-esophageal reflux (reflux of food between stomach and esophagus).

Diagnosis of asthma

The diagnosis of asthma is largely based on the history of the patient, as there is **no specific test** or marker for asthma. However, the demonstration of reversible airway obstruction on pulmonary function testing (impossible to perform in young children, but feasible from the ages of five to six years) in older children is a further confirmation of the diagnosis.

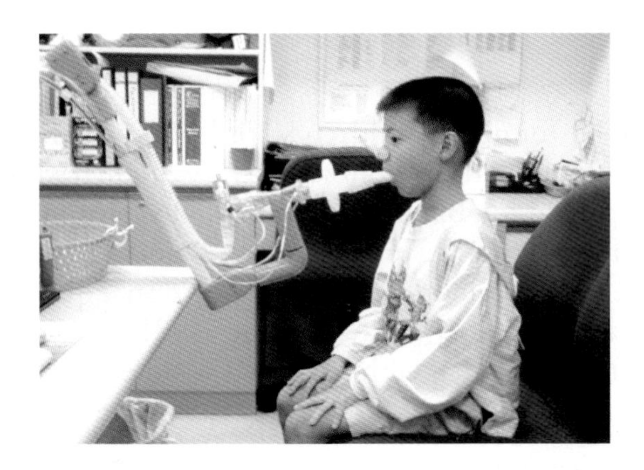

Fig. 5 Lung function testing. Lung function testing is an important tool in the global assessment of asthma severity. Furthermore, results of lung function testing show data on lung growth (which can be impaired as a result of severe asthma) and have a prognostic value, as severe lung function abnormalities are a risk for the development of adult asthma.

A history of recurrent wheezing and/or chronic cough is likely to be asthma, unless proven otherwise. The diagnosis is usually made after three attacks or after chronic symptoms of at least one month.

Clinical examination can be totally normal, especially in-between attacks. Hence, the lack of physical signs does not exclude a diagnosis of asthma. Symptoms that can be present are: an abnormal lung auscultation (wheezing, rales), and in cases of severe past attacks, malformations of the chest can be seen (Harrison's sulci – see picture in Chapter1).

Children with allergic BA can also show other symptoms of allergy, such as eczema, allergic rhinitis (congested nose, runny nose, itchy nose, sneezing) and allergic conjunctivitis (red, itchy eyes). The diagnosis of BA is largely based on history and clinical examination. However, additional tests, such as lung function testing and allergy testing, will enable a better insight on severity and cause of the underlying BA.

Lung function testing (Fig. 5)

Abnormalities in lung function

can be found in children with BA. However, no abnormality is specific for BA, and can also be found in other lung diseases. The most common abnormalities of the lung function that can be found in children with BA are:

1. Decreased lung growth as a consequence of ongoing asthma
2. Bronchial obstruction, which is reversible after administration of a bronchodilator (beta-agonist)
3. Ongoing inflammation, which can be detected by an increase of exhaled nitric oxide (eNO) (e.g. a marker of inflammation)
4. Bronchial hyperreactivity, which can be demonstrated by inhaling histamine or methacholine

For most lung function testing, it is necessary that the child is cooperative. Usually, lung function testing can be performed from the ages of five to seven years. Special lung function testing is now available for young, non-cooperative children.

Allergy testing

Assessment of an underlying allergy is important in children with BA, because allergy can determine the prognosis, as children who are very allergic tend to have more persistent asthma, and also because of therapeutic consequences (avoidance of allergens). Allergy can be detected using two techniques (for more details see Chapter 11 on diagnostic testing):

1. Detection of the allergic antibodies (IgE) in the blood using a specific immunological test.
2. Skin prick testing (Fig. 6). Skin prick testing is most commonly performed on the forearm, although the back is sometimes used. The arm is first cleaned with alcohol, following which a drop of commercially-produced allergen extract is placed onto a marked area of skin. Using a sterile lancet, a small prick through the drop is made. This allows a small amount of allergen to enter the skin. If the child is allergic, a small mosquito-like lump will appear at the site of testing over 15-20 minutes. Skin tests are well tolerated and accurate, even in small children and infants. Skin prick testing is the test of choice in allergy, because it is cheaper and more sensitive than determination of IgE in the blood.

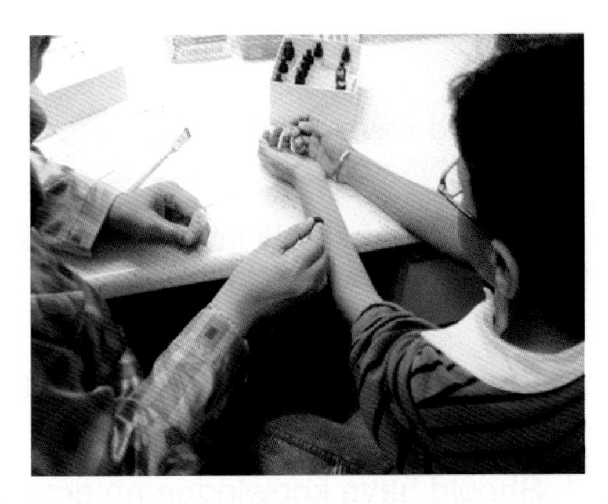

Fig. 6 Skin prick testing. Allergy testing (skin prick testing) in asthma gives information on the possibility of underlying allergic triggers, such as the house dust mite, and the results have a prognostic value: children with severe underlying allergy tend more to develop persistent asthma.

Treatment of asthma

Asthma in children is a non-curable disease (or syndrome) with a variable, even unpredictable evolution: some children will spontaneously grow out of it, while others will suffer from persistent asthma for the rest of their lives. Usually, persistence of BA is associated with a bad lung function and/or with severe allergy. The good news, however, is that symptoms of asthma are controllable in most children, because of the availability of effective and safe anti-asthmatic medications. However, once the treatment is stopped, re-occurrence of BA is the rule, as most treatments have no carry-over effect (except for immunotherapy, which can have a sustained effect, but not in all patients).

Treating asthma is more than just prescribing medication. It is offering the child and the family a whole package of information on BA, now referred to as **a holistic approach**, including educating the child and discussing

1. Should have basic knowledge on asthma.

2. Should be closely involved in the management of the child.

3. Should be able to recognize asthma symptoms

4. Should have knowledge on acute treatment (through an action plan)and on maintenance treatment.

Fig. 7 Involvement of parents. Treating asthma is more than prescribing medications. It is a global approach to the child and the whole family.

appropriate interventions, such as the administration of anti-asthmatic medication. **Appropriate education of the child (Fig. 7) and the family is pivotal in the treatment of BA**. Goals of asthma treatment include: control of all asthma symptoms, prevention of new asthma attacks, and allowing the child to lead a healthy normal life. Recent guidelines on the management of BA now focus more on achieving control of asthma, using individualized management plans in the context of a team effort that includes the patient, relevant family members or care takers, doctor, nurse/clinic assistant, and pharmacist.

Control of BA is defined as the control of several outcomes, including:

- No daytime symptoms (twice or less per week)
- No limitation of daily activities, including exercise
- No nocturnal symptoms or awakening because of BA
- No need for reliever treatment (twice or less per week)

- No exacerbations
- Normal or near-normal lung function results

Table 2 shows the different aspects of treatment of bronchial asthma. The treatment should be individually tailored, depending on type, severity, and prognosis of the child's BA.

Asthma medications

There are two groups of asthma medications:

1. Relievers. To treat symptoms. Usually these medications open the airways and are also called bronchodilators. They are only used when the child has symptoms, and they have no effect upon the long-term outcome of BA (Table 3).

Table 2 The Different Aspects of the Treatment of Bronchial Asthma

1. Education (child + family) and self-assessment and management
2. Avoidance of all triggers (allergens, irritants)
3. Medication (preventers - relievers)
4. Immunotherapy (specific cases)
5. Other
   - sports
   - treatment of upper airways abnormalities (rhinitis, sinusitis, etc.)
   - treatment of gastro-esophageal reflux (especially in infants)

Table 3 Relievers

Class of Medication	Route of Delivery	Common Examples
Short-acting beta-agonists	Inhaled	Salbutamol (Ventolin) Terbutaline (Bricanyl)
	Oral	Salbutamol (Ventolin) Terbutaline (Bricanyl)
Anti-cholinergics	Inhaled	Ipratropium bromide (Atrovent)
Corticosteroids	Oral or injected	Prednisolone Hydrocortisone

2. Preventers. To prevent new symptoms by reducing the degree of inflammation (e.g. anti-inflammatory agents) (Table 4). These medications will control asthma, allowing the child to have a higher change to grow out of BA. These medications should be taken on a daily basis, and long-term administration is necessary to control the underlying inflammation (some children need to take their preventers for many years). The most common preventer is *an inhaled corticosteroid*, which is now the treatment of first choice for most asthmatic children. Inhaled corticosteroids in **normal dose** are very effective and safe: virtually no side effects have been described, and these medications have now been used in millions of asthmatic children during the last 40 years. Other forms of preventers, such as leukotriene-receptor antagonists (LTRA) can be taken orally, but are usually less effective than inhaled corticosteroids. Long-acting beta-agonists (LABA) can also be used, but only in combination with an inhaled corticosteroid as an add-on treatment, which can be useful in a minority of older asthmatic children with severe underlying asthma. LABA should not be used in young children (<5 years), because of the lack of sufficient safety data.

Table 4 Preventers

Class of Medication	Route of Delivery	Common Examples
Inhaled corticosteroids	Inhaled	Beclomethasone dipropionate (Becotide, Beclo-asthma) Budesonide (Pulmicort, Inflammide) Fluticasone propionate (Flixotide) Ciclesonide
Leukotriene-receptor-antagonists (LTRA)	Oral	Montelukast (Singulair)
Long-acting beta-agonists (LABA)	Inhaled	Salmeterol (Seretide = in combination with fluticasone dipropionate) Formoterol (Symbicort = in combination with budesonide)

The first choice preventive medication in asthma is an inhaled corticosteroid. These medications are very effective in preventing asthma symptoms and have an excellent safety profile.

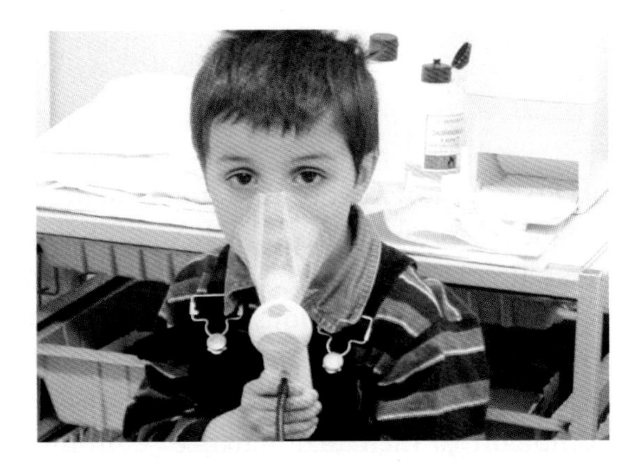

Fig. 8 Boy with acute asthma attack. Nebulizer to treat an acute or severe attack of asthma.

Treatment of acute asthma-attacks

Usually, acute symptoms of BA are treated with relievers (Fig. 8), especially with short-acting beta-agonists, such as salbutamol (Ventolin). However, sometimes symptoms can be severe, needing more treatment than beta-agonists, and some children need to be admitted to a hospital. Severe attacks usually

A general rule for parents of asthmatic children:

If the reliever medication seems to be non-effective (symptoms persist despite administration of the reliever), it means the attack needs more intensive treatment and it is advisable to get medical help without wasting precious time!

occur in children who were not diagnosed as suffering from BA (first attack), in young children with certain viral infections of the lower airways (RSV infections), or in asthmatic children who are not compliant to their maintenance treatment. Symptoms of acute BA include shortness of breath, cough, wheezing or chest tightness, or a combination of these symptoms. The speed of progression of acute symptoms is variable and can be anything from a few minutes to a few hours or days. Often, perception of the severity of acute symptoms by patients, relatives, or even by health care workers is poor, and this may result in underestimation of the severity of an acute attack. Therefore, assessment of the severity of the acute symptoms is important. The child and family must be familiar with the acute action plan and act on the earliest sign of deterioration before the attack requires emergency care or hospitalization.

Treatment in the hospital includes administration of oxygen, high doses of corticosteroids, and intra-venous administration of theophylline or beta-agonists. In severe attacks, leading to respiratory insufficiency, intubation and mechanical ventilation might be necessary.

Administration of inhaler medications

In most children, anti-asthmatic medications are administered directly into the lower airways,

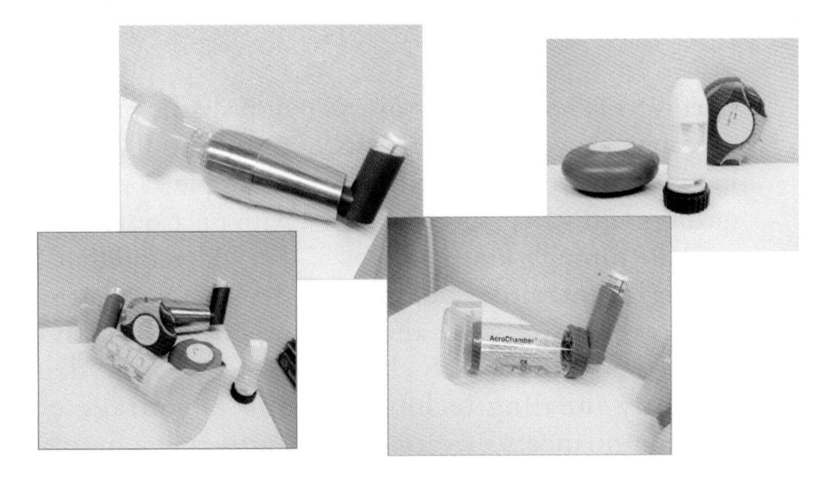

Fig. 9 Devices and holding chambers.

using different inhaler devices. Success of treatment is very much dependent on the correct choice of inhaler device and the prescription of an appropriate holding chamber device (also called a "spacer") when necessary, mainly according to the age of the asthmatic child. It is also very important to educate the child and the caregivers on the use of the inhaler device and ask them to demonstrate the procedure to affirm that learning has occurred, and to optimize intra-bronchial administration of the medications. The following recommendations in choosing an inhaler device and holding chamber (Fig. 9) can be put forward:

1. For children below four years: Metered dose inhaler (puffer – MDI) with spacer and face mask.
2. For children aged four to six years: MDI with spacer with mouthpiece
3. For children beyond six years: MDI with spacer with mouthpiece or dry powder inhaler (such as Accuhaler or Turbuhaler).

Monitoring of asthma management

Monitoring of BA treatment is very important for a number of reasons, such as, assessment of asthma evolution and asthma severity (childhood BA can be very dynamic, showing spontaneous improvement or deterioration), quality of life (sleep, sports), lung growth (through lung function testing), general development of the child (growth) and to adapt the treatment, to check regularly inhaling technique and compliance to treatment. Therefore, all children with BA who are on a maintenance treatment should be in follow-up with a medical doctor, and those with severe asthma might need specialized medical care (pediatrician, pediatric allergist, or pediatric pulmonologist). The treatment of BA should be kept as simple as possible, preferably with once or twice a day dosing. For older children, new inhaler devices, e.g. turbuhalers and other breath-activated devices may enhance drug delivery and encourage compliance. Furthermore, regular assessment of lung function, especially of lung growth, is useful in adapting the treatment. Repeated allergy testing (yearly) can be indicated, assessing whether or not the child is growing out of the underlying allergy.

Prognosis of childhood BA

BA in children is a dynamic disease and a large number of children will grow out of it. The underlying mechanisms of "growing out" are fairly unknown: it seems that the child's lungs become less responsive to the external triggers. A number of children keep having positive allergy testing, but are no longer sensitive to the underlying allergy. Usually, young children with viral-induced asthma (no underlying allergy) tend to grow out of their BA around the ages of five to seven years. In contrast, children with allergic BA tend to have persistence of their symptoms up to puberty. During puberty, however, about 50% of them will grow out of their BA, but in some cases BA can re-occur during early adulthood and persist for many years.

In a study from New Zealand, in which more than 600 children were followed for wheezing up till adulthood (mean age: 26 years), the following was shown:

1. 14.5% have persistent BA from childhood into adulthood
2. 12.4% grow out of BA, but relapse during early adulthood
3. 15% completely grow out of their asthma
4. 9.5% still have infrequent wheezing during adulthood
5. 21.2% have BA, but only during childhood
6. 27.4% never had any symptoms of asthma

The authors concluded that BA (wheezing) is a common symptom, but it is often mild and transient. Of the study members, 72.6% had reported wheezing during at least one assessment by the age of 26 years, and 51.4% had reported such wheezing at more than one assessment.

Long-term follow-up studies from the Netherlands and Australia showed similar results: about 50% of children with allergic BA will continue to have symptoms during adulthood.

From these different studies, it was concluded that the factors associated with a bad prognosis (e.g. not growing out of BA) are:

1. A disturbed lung function
2. High airway hyperresponsiveness
3. Female sex
4. Smoking
5. Early onset of BA
6. Allergy, especially house dust mite sensitization

In asthmatic children receiving immunotherapy (subcutaneous immunotherapy or sublingual immunotherapy) the long-term prognosis becomes better, as it was shown that immunotherapy can have an important carry-over effect, helping the child to grow out of BA. Improving the lung function by sports might also have a positive impact upon prognosis, but more studies on this subject are needed.

5

Allergy of upper airways (allergic rhinitis and allergic rhino-sinusitis) and eyes (allergic conjunctivitis)

Introduction

The most common allergic disease in children and adults is allergy of the nose, called allergic **rhinitis** (AR). If the sinuses are also involved, the term **rhino-sinusitis** is used. In a number of children, AR occurs in association with allergic symptoms of the eyes, also referred to as **allergic conjunctivitis**. When both nose and eyes are involved, the term allergic **rhino-conjunctivitis** is used.

AR affects more than 30% of older children in Singapore, and is mainly caused and maintained by an underlying allergy to house dust mites. In young children, however, rhinitis is also very common, but it is usually a non-allergic condition, caused by sensitive upper airways and triggered by viral infections. This

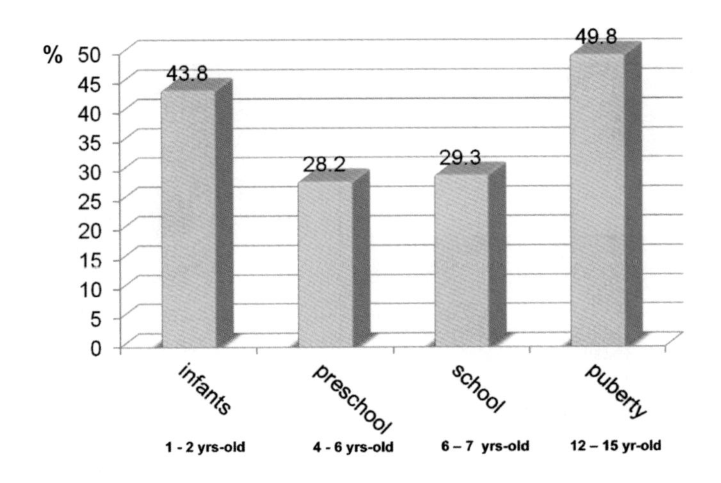

Fig. 1 Prevalence of rhinitis in Singaporean children (own data).

occurs especially in children attending day-care centers (i.e. children having close contact with many other children), which can result in the so-called back-to-back infections of the upper airways. In our own studies on two-year-old children, we found that more than 40% suffered from chronic rhinitis. However, most of these children were non-allergic (negative SPT), and only symptoms of rhino-conjunctivitis in young children (which is uncommon) were associated with an underlying allergy.

The prevalence of AR (Fig. 1) is increasing and underreporting probably occurs worldwide. Many people consider it **normal** for children to have a blocked or runny nose, and they use the term "normal blocked or runny nose". However, underdiagnosis and undertreatment of AR can lead to severe morbidity (complications) (see below).

The number of children affected by AR has doubled in the past 20 years. As a result, roughly one-third of all individuals currently affected are ≤ 17 years of age worldwide. According to the ISAAC studies, AR affects 0.8% to 14.9% of six- to seven-year-olds and 1.4% to 39.7% of 13- to 14-year-olds. Socioeconomic costs of AR are considerable. In children aged ≥ 12 years, direct US expenditures (e.g. physician's visits, medications) in 1996 amounted $2.3 billion.

1

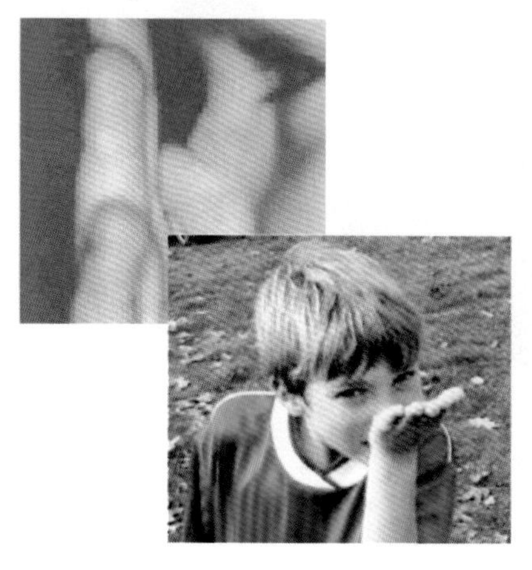

2

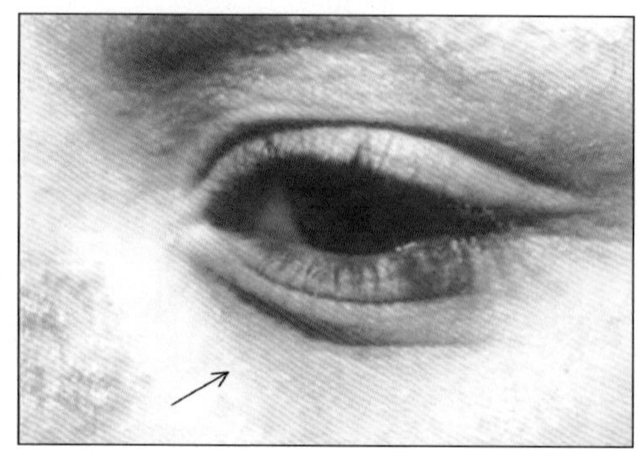

Fig. 2 Allergic salute and allergic shiners. Signs of allergic rhinitis 1. allergic salute 2. allergic shiners: dark area's under the eyes, also referred to as Dennie-Morgan fields, which are a consequence of congestion of sinuses.

Symptoms of AR and clinical entities

Major symptoms of AR include blocked nose, runny nose, itchy nose, and sneezing. However, none of these symptoms are specific, and other causes of rhinitis, such as infections (colds, flu) or irritations (by smoke or perfumes) of the nose can lead to similar symptoms. Symptoms of AR can be chronic (perennial) in the case of chronic exposure to the allergen (for instance exposure to house dust mites), or seasonal in the case of allergy to seasonal occurring allergens, such as different pollen. In tropical areas, however, seasonal AR is uncommon, because of the lack of a specific pollen season.

The more specific symptoms for AR are itchy nose and sneezing. In the case of an underlying house dust mite allergy, these symptoms occur more often during early morning or immediately after waking up. A typical sign of AR is the so-called "allergic salute," (Fig. 2) being a consequence of the itchy nose, and leading to the presence of a horizontal line on the nose. Another sign of AR is the so-called allergic shiners

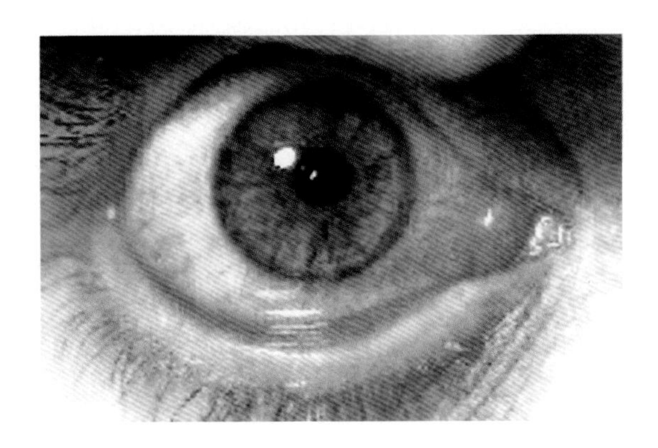

Fig. 3 Severe conjunctivitis. The eye is red, swollen, itchy and tearing. Rubbing of the eye may lead to secondary infection.

under the eyes, being a sign of venous congestion from paranasal sinuses, suggesting sinusitis.

Clinical examination of the child can be completely normal, but can also reveal the following signs:

1. Allergic shiners (dark areas under the eyes)
2. Horizontal line on the nose, as a consequence of the allergic salute
3. A swollen, wet, and grey-pale nasal mucosa
4. In cases of a postnasal drip, mucus can be seen in the throat, which can lead to the so-called "throat cough."

Entities that are related to AR are the allergic rhino-sinusitis (involvement of sinuses) and the allergic rhino-conjunctivitis (involvement of the conjunctiva of the eyes), which were already partially covered in Chapter 1.

As a reminder:

- **Rhino-conjunctivitis** (Fig. 3) is a typical manifestation of allergy, usually to pets or pollen (far less to house dust mites). Symptoms include rhinitis and eye symptoms (redness, itch, tearing). Blinking can be the only manifestation of conjunctivitis. In rare cases, conjunctivitis can be very severe, affecting the cornea of the eye. This is the so-called kerato-conjunctivitis. Rhino-conjunctivitis should always be treated to avoid complications, such as keratitis (inflammation of the cornea), ocular perforation,

1. **It is important to treat all children with AR, in order to avoid a large number of complications (see text for details).**
2. **A normal blocked nose does not exist!**

keratoconus, opacities of the cornea, and cataract.

- **Rhino-sinusitis** is suspected when the symptoms of AR are associated with excessive production of mucus, leading to postnasal dripping and the so-called "throat cough." Chronic rhino-sinusitis has to be distinguished from acute rhino-sinusitis, the latter being an acute bacterial infection of the sinuses that causes symptoms of pain and fever, and of which the mechanisms are similar to those of acute otitis.

The effects of AR are often underestimated and the disease is often unjustly considered trivial (Fig. 4). A large number of children

1. Medical complications
   - infections (otitis, sinusitis)
   - hypertrophic adenoids
     (→ more infections and sleep apnea syndrome)
   - risk for asthma
2. Non-medical complications
   - bad sleep, bad school results
   - psychological problems and isolation

Fig. 4 Complications of allergic rhinitis.

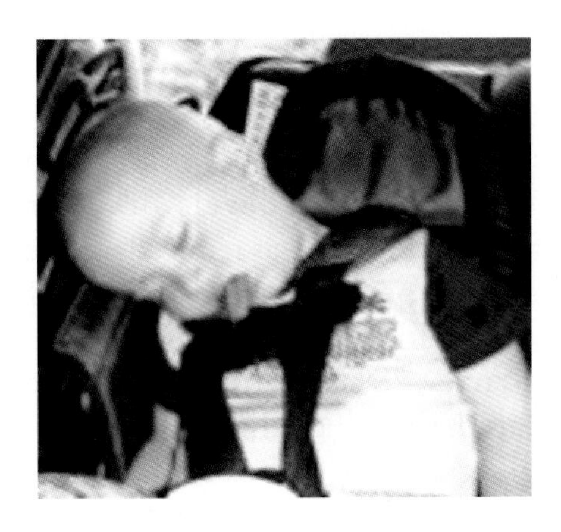

Fig. 5 Sleeping child. Children with undertreated allergic rhinitis are drowsy, tired and become isolated.

with AR accept living with their symptoms, consider it "normal," and don't ask for medical advice. However, evidence indicates that the symptoms of AR can have considerable deleterious effects on schoolchildren (Fig. 5), including sleep abnormalities (i.e. obstructive sleep apnea syndrome or OSAS), increased school absenteeism, cognitive impairment, poor school performance, and behavioral and psychological problems. Another major concern is that underdiagnosis and inadequate treatment of AR increases the risk of serious comorbid conditions, such as bronchial asthma (BA). In a number of studies it was shown that appropriate treatment of AR prevents the development of BA. Furthermore, the obvious link between AR and associated conditions of the upper airways such as chronic rhino-sinusitis, nasal polyps, recurrent throat infections (pharyngitis), adenoid hypertrophy, tubal dysfunction, and otitis media with effusion or laryngitis are additional reasons to treat rhinitis optimally.

What are the children's complaints?

Apart from the classical symptoms, allergic children often complain about difficulty in concentrating. Most of them report decreased cognitive processing, slowed thinking, reduced ability to remember, and difficulty sustaining attention during allergy seasons. Furthermore, AR goes along with daytime sleepiness, difficulty staying awake, a worn-out feeling, higher levels of mental fatigue, as well as reduced motivation, perhaps as a result of sleep disturbances. In one recent survey, 78% of participants indicated they had difficulty obtaining a good night's sleep, 75% had difficulty getting to sleep, and 64% awakened during the night. The impact of AR is also significant at the emotional level: over one-third of patients feel irritable, frustrated, and stressed. Self-esteem may be compromised, as many adolescents with AR report being embarrassed by their symptoms and appearance. Symptoms of AR may limit interaction with peers.

Fatigue and allergy

The traditional view is that fatigue and depressed feelings are the result of the physical effects of the illness or side effects of allergy medications. Allergic rhinitis can, by itself, introduce significant sedation, and daytime sleepiness is related to the severity of the disease. Also, sedation was the most troublesome side effect of certain older medications used to treat AR in the past, occurring in up to 55% of patients. In children, the sedating effect of first-generation antihistamines is implicated in impairing school performance, cognitive function, and productivity. Other side effects of first-generation antihistamines include somnolence, drowsiness, decreased alertness or restlessness, nervousness, and insomnia. Therefore, the older antihistamines, although effective on symptoms, are not used anymore in the treatment of AR.

However, according to the affected patients, the most important problem related to their condition is the **impairment of sleep quality**. The severity of AR significantly influences the mean duration of nocturnal sleep during the week and weekends, the frequency of daytime sleepiness, and the time necessary to fall asleep. Sleep is significantly more impaired in patients with severe AR than in those with the mild type. Recent research has suggested that daytime somnolence in AR can be attributed to chronic inflammation of the nasal mucosa, leading to nasal congestion and obstructed nasal passageways, and resulting in disturbed sleep.

Several studies have shown the relationship among nasal obstruction and abnormal breathing during sleep, snoring, and sleep apnea. In fact, allergic patients with nasal congestion

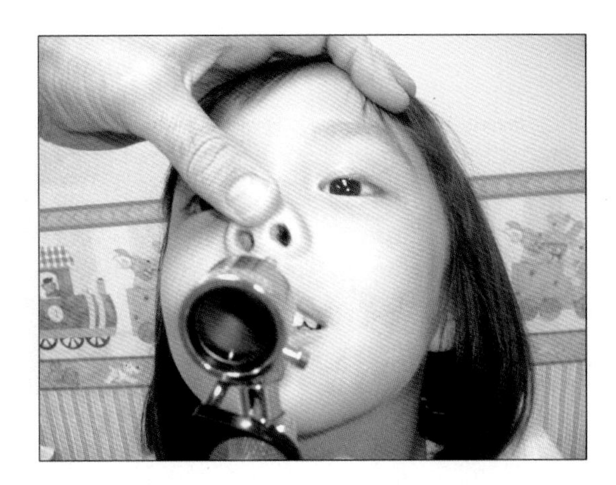

Fig. 6 Looking into the nose. Clinical examination of a child with rhinitis includes a so-called "rhinoscopia anterior," which means "a look in the nose." By looking in the nose it is possible to diagnose the existence of rhinitis. In case of persistent allergy, as a cause of rhinitis, the mucosa will be swollen, pale and grey. Furthermore, sometimes pus can be seen, coming from the sinuses. By looking in the throat it is possible to see postnasal dripping, suggesting involvement of sinuses.

had 1.8 times greater chance of moderate-to-severe sleep-disordered breathing than those without congestion. Snoring occurred in 28% of a large group of non-selected children, and habitual, daily snoring was present in 6%. Snoring scores were associated with higher levels of inattention and hyperactivity. Obstructive apneas were longer and more frequent in patients with AR with nasal obstruction than in those without obstruction when sleep was measured by means of polysomnography. Compared with healthy control subjects, patients with AR had 10 times more micro-arousals from sleep. Micro-arousals can ultimately lead to daytime fatigue due to the associated sleep fragmentation.

Diagnosis of AR

The diagnosis of AR, rhino-conjunctivitis, and rhino-sinusitis is based on the history and the clinical examination (Fig. 6) of

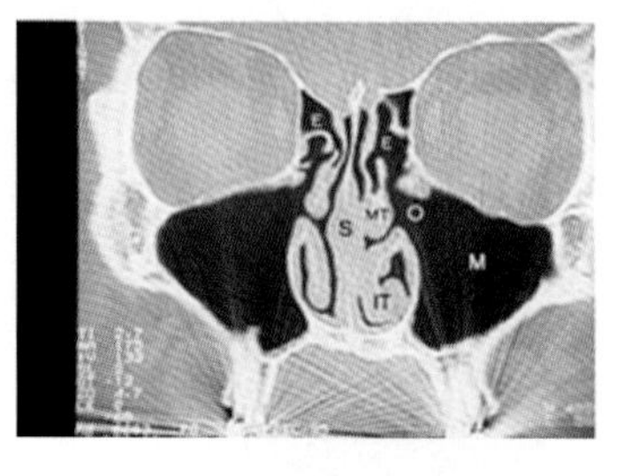

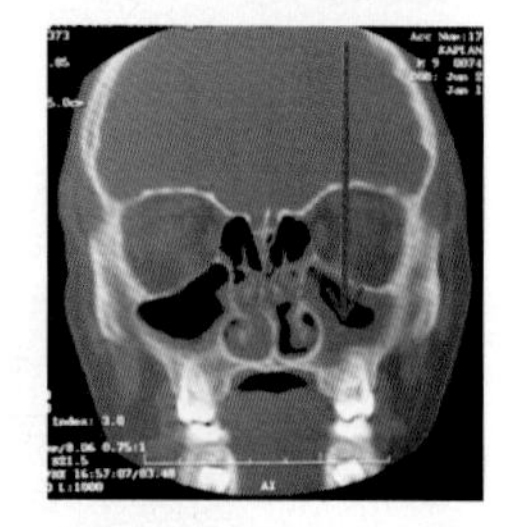

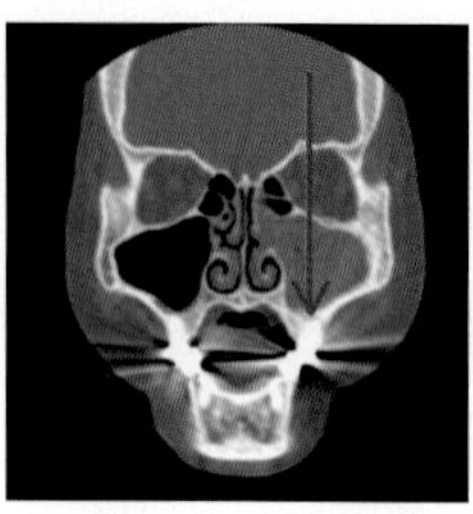

Acute sinusitis: the sinus is filled with pus

Fig. 7 CAT-scan of chronic sinusitis. In theory, a CT-scan is better for diagnosing sinusitis than an X-ray. However, in most children the diagnosis can be made based on clinical grounds, and therefore, most children do not need imaging of sinuses.

the patient, and is confirmed by allergy testing (skin prick testing or determination of specific IgE in the blood). Usually, no other tests are necessary in most children with symptoms of AR.

In exceptional cases of persistent or severe rhino-sinusitis, imaging of the paranasal sinuses can be considered, such as X-ray or CT-scan (Fig. 7).

In cases of severe conjunctivitis a detailed ophthalmological assessment is desirable, including a check-up of the severity and extension of conjunctivitis and assessment of affection of the eye (i.e. kerato-conjunctivitis).

Treatment

It is generally accepted that **all allergic diseases of the upper airways** (rhinitis, rhino-sinusitis) and the eyes (conjunctivitis) should be treated, not only to avoid complications, but also because of the positive impact of treatment on the child's quality of life. In a number of well-designed studies, it was shown that treating AR improves dramatically the

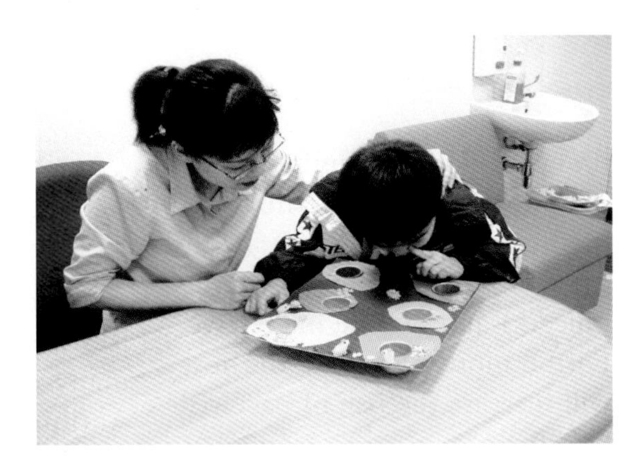

Fig. 8 Child learning to blow the nose. A trained nurse is teaching a child how to blow the nose, by playing a game, called" blow the frogs in the pool with your nose".

quality of sleep and learning abilities.

1. Treatment of allergic rhinitis

The treatment of AR is made up of three parts:

1. **Allergen avoidance + avoidance of other irritants**
2. **Cleaning of the nose** (i.e. teaching the child how to blow the nose (Fig. 8), especially before administration of intra-nasal medication)
3. **Administration of medication** (antihistamines - intranasal corticosteroids)

Other treatments that can have a role in children with severe AR are the leukotriene receptor antagonists (such as montelukast), disodium cromoglycate (DSCG), and immunotherapy (mainly sublingual immunotherapy (SLIT)). The role of other immunomodulatory treatments still needs to be explored. Pro-, pre-, and synbiotics, which are now increasingly used to prevent or treat allergies, have not been shown to be effective in children with AR.

As part of the treatment, it is very important to teach the child to keep the nose as clean as possible, by teaching him or her how to blow the nose and by advising the use of saline water (sea water) for this purpose. When children are prescribed intranasal medication, it is especially important to clean the nose before the administration of the medication. If not, the medication will not reach the nasal mucosa (sticks into the phlegm) and will be ineffective. Furthermore, phlegm in the nose will increase the risk of bacterial infections.

Medication for AR constitutes two major groups of medicines: **antihistamines**, which are taken orally as a tablet or syrup (some can also be administrated intra-nasally), and **intranasal corticosteroids**, which are administrated directly in the nose. Both groups of mediations are effective in the treatment of AR, and both groups have an excellent safety profile, even in very young children. Treatment with intranasal corticosteroids or antihistamines has been shown to reduce nasal obstruction (congestion) and to improve sleep. Furthermore, treatment reduces daytime sleepiness, daytime fatigue, and sleep problems. Treatment with the newer non-sedating antihistamines can significantly improve the learning capacity in children with AR, and when compared to a placebo, the new antihistamines reduce absenteeism and classroom impairment.

* **Antihistamines:**

Histamine is one of the major mediators released during symptoms of AR. Therefore, histamine is the cause of many of the symptoms of AR. Antihistamines block the effect of histamine by (competitive) binding on the histamine receptors of the cellular membranes, thereby preventing cellular activation that leads to allergic symptoms.

Antihistamines can help relieve the following symptoms: itching, sneezing, and nasal discharge. Some newer antihistamines also reduce nasal congestion. Antihistamines, however, have no or only very little effect on symptoms of asthma or eczema. If possible, patients should take antihistamines *before* an anticipated allergy attack of AR or before exposure to the allergens. Therefore, in cases of house dust mite allergy, antihistamines should be taken in the evening, as the exposure to house dust mites is highest during the night. In cases of pollen allergy, it is advisable to take antihistamines in the morning.

Many antihistamines are available. They include short-acting and long-acting forms and are available as tablets and syrups. Others are available as nasal-inhalers or eye drops.

Antihistamines are generally categorized as **first- and second-generation**. First-generation antihistamines may cause side effects, such as drowsiness, which is much less the case with

First-Generation Antihistamines include diphenhydramine, carbinoxamine, clemastine, chlorpheniramine, brompheniramine, ketotifen, and promethazine.

It is important to note that these antihistamines should never be used for children younger than age two, because, in rare cases, they may cause life-threatening breathing problems.

Side Effects of first-generation antihistamines include:

- Drowsiness and impaired thinking
- Dry mouth
- Dizziness
- Agitation
- Insomnia or nightmares
- Sore throat
- Rapid heart beat and chest tightness (uncommon and should be reported)

Second-Generation (= non-sedating) Antihistamines

The newer second-generation antihistamines do not usually cause drowsiness to the extent that the first generation antihistamines do. Therefore, they are sometimes referred to collectively as non-sedating antihistamines. The second-generation drugs include loratadine, desloratidine, cetirizine, levocetirizine, and fexofenadine.

Cetirizine and loratidine have been approved for young children. Both medications have an excellent safety profile in young children and are effective in AR and urticaria (not in eczema). Cetirizine is the only antihistamine approved for both indoor and outdoor allergies and for infants as young as six months. Both are available in syrup form. Studies with cetirizine have reported fewer symptoms in children allergic to dust mites, and one study reported that infants with allergies who were given cetirizine were much less likely to develop asthma later on than untreated infants. At this time, loratidine is generally the preferred drug for young people because it has the least negative effect on concentration and learning. Women who are pregnant or nursing should avoid these medications unless recommended by a doctor.

Young children hate intranasal medication. Parents have to "fight" with their child to administer the medication, and this leads to low treatment compliance.

Side Effects and Precautions

- Common side effects include headache, dry mouth, and dry nose. (These are often only temporary and go away during treatment.)
- Drowsiness occurs in about 10% of adults and between 2-4% of children.
- Uncommon side effects include rapid heart beat and chest tightness. Tell your doctor if these effects occur.
- Extended-release forms of loratadine and cetirizine have other ingredients that can cause other symptoms, including nervousness, restlessness, and insomnia.

Nasal-Spray

Antihistamines, such as azelastine and levocabastine are available in nasal spray form and have a good safety profile in children. They can reduce nasal congestion as well as allergy symptoms. Both reduce symptoms, although azelastine may be more effective in some patients. Their disadvantages are a bitter taste, drowsiness, and expense. They are not as effective as steroid nasal sprays.

Combinations of Antihistamines and Decongestants

Many prescription and non-prescription products that combine antihistamines and decongestants are available and are sold over-the-counter. Usually, these combinations have no major advantages compared to antihistamines and should be avoided in all children!

The first choice treatment for AR in young children is a second generation antihistamine that has extensive efficacy and safety data in that age group. Medications such as cetirizine and levocetirizine

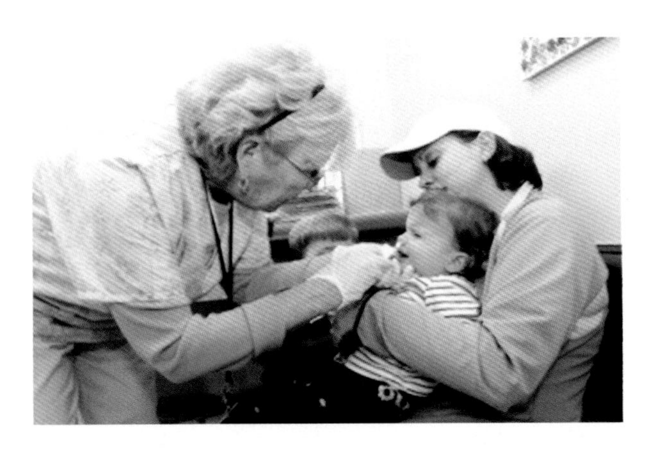

Fig. 9 Most young children don't like intra-nasal medication and parents sometimes need to fight with the child to administer the medication.

fulfill these criteria, and are now the first choice treatments for AR in young children. Data on loratidine and desloratidine are less extensive, while other antihistamines have not been studied in young children (except for limited and older studies with ketotifen).

Intranasal corticosteroids

Intra-nasal corticosteroids are effective and safe to treat AR in children, even in young children. However, young children dislike very much intranasal sprays, which will substantially affect compliance to intranasal sprays.

Intranasal corticosteroids such as beclomethasone dipropionate, budesonide, and fluticasone have been extensively studied in children and no major side effects have been reported. These medications have a better effect on chronic symptoms of AR, as they are able to suppress ongoing inflammation (in contrast to antihistamines, which are more suitable for acute attacks of AR). In cases of severe AR, antihistamines and intranasal corticosteroids are combined. With this combination of drugs (plus allergen avoidance and appropriate nose cleaning), most children with AR can be sufficiently treated.

If symptoms persist, despite this approach, other possible treatments to add on to this treatment include:

Never administer a cough syrup to infants or to children with asthma

a. Montelukast

In a limited number of studies in children with AR, a mild to moderate effect of montelukast was shown. Therefore, it was suggested that montelukast can be used as an "add-on" treatment for those children with severe AR in whom the symptoms persist despite treatment with antihistamines and intranasal corticosteroids. However, montelukast is still not a first choice treatment for AR: its effectiveness is not superior compared to antihistamines, and montelukast is also more expensive than antihistamines.

b. Immunotherapy (see also Chapter 11)

Immunotherapy is an old treatment that has been reappraised recently, especially because of the availability of a sublingual (i.e. administration under the tongue) type of immunotherapy, also referred to as SLIT. Immunotherapy means the administration of standardized increasing amounts of a specific allergen, in order to desensitize (or hyposensitize) the patient to that allergen. In earlier days, subcutaneous administration was used, which was painful and which could induce potential side effects. In contrast, SLIT is very child friendly, can be given at home, and is not associated with major side effects.

In different studies on SLIT it was shown that SLIT has its highest effectiveness in patients with AR or allergic rhino-conjunctivitis, especially in those children who are allergic to pollen, and also in those allergic to house dust mites. SLIT is less effective in asthma and eczema. Disadvantages of SLIT are its cost and the fact that the duration of the treatment to achieve a long-term effect is at least three years, and in some children, five years. The advantage of SLIT is that it can make the child less allergic and that the

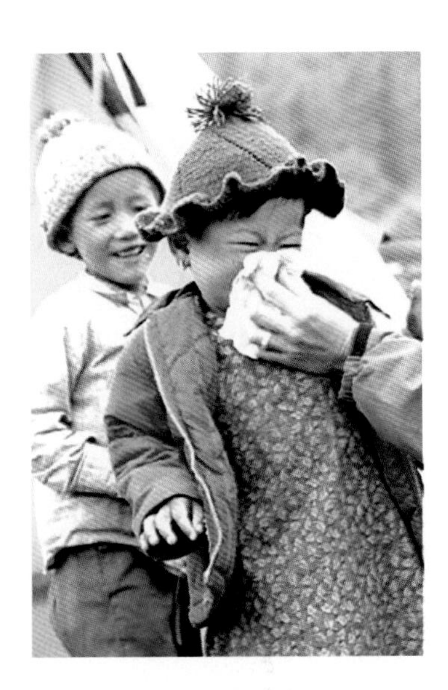

Fig. 10 Blowing the nose. Keeping the nose clean is essential in the treatment of rhinitis. This will reduce the risk of infections of the nose (colds, flu) and will also allow intra-nasal medication to reach better the mucosa of the nose, resulting in higher effectiveness. In contrast, "sucking up" the phlegm will increase the risk of sinusitis.

effect persists for many years, even after having stopped the SLIT.

2. Treatment of allergic rhino-sinusitis

Treatment of allergic rhino-sinusitis is very similar of that of allergic rhinitis: allergen avoidance and the usage of antihistamines and intra-nasal corticosteroids. Treatment of allergic rhino-sinusitis, however, *should be more intense*, focusing on removing secretions (i.e. cleaning of the nose) (Fig. 10) in order to avoid potential complications (such as

GENERAL CONCLUSION

Allergies of upper airways and eyes are very common, and can induce significant morbidity, which might lead to severe complications. Therefore, it is important that every child with an allergic disease of the upper airways and/or eyes is treated optimally. Treatment will avoid complications and improve the quality of life considerably, including school results and quality of sleep.

acute bacterial infections). The child should be very well taught to clean the nose and to remove all phlegm. In cases of postnasal dripping of phlegm, causing a typical throat cough and throat clearing, a cough syrup might be used to improve sleep, but never to infants and never in cases of concomitant asthma. In infants, cough syrup may suppress normal breathing, and has been associated with sudden infant death syndrome (SIDS), while in asthmatic children, cough syrups can mask the asthmatic symptoms, which may lead to increased severity of asthma.

In rare cases of chronic rhinosinusitis, with thick phlegm and postnasal dripping, a short course of nebulizer treatment, administrating saline or medications that can reduce phlegm production (such as anticholinergics), might be justified in order to reduce the thickness of the phlegm.

3. Treatment of allergic conjunctivitis

Allergic conjunctivitis should always be treated, to avoid complications affecting the eyes. Standard treatment includes antihistamines and eye drops containing corticosteroids or disodium cromoglycate (DSCG). DSCG is a mild anti-inflammatory medication that blocks mast cells without side effects. The drug can be safely administered for long periods.

In cases of severe allergic conjunctivitis involving also the eye (i.e. keratoconjunctivitis), an extensive ophthalmological check-up is necessary. A more intense treatment includes the usage of local immunomodulators, such as cyclosporine, and the usage of immunotherapy (SLIT).

6 Eczema or Atopic Dermatitis

Introduction

Eczema is now considered as a group of chronic skin diseases of which **allergic eczema or atopic dermatitis (AD)** is the most common type in children. Other types of childhood eczema include **seborrhoeic eczema** and **contact dermatitis**. Moreover, a distinction between atopic eczema and **constitutional (or intrinsic)** eczema can also be made, referring to the presence or absence of an underlying allergy. In infants from allergic families without evidence of an underlying allergy (but who are expected to become allergic after prolonged exposure to allergens), the term **pre-allergic eczema** can be used. Recently, it was proposed that the nomenclature on eczema should be revised and that the term AD should be replaced by **atopic eczema/dermatitis syndrome (AEDS)**.

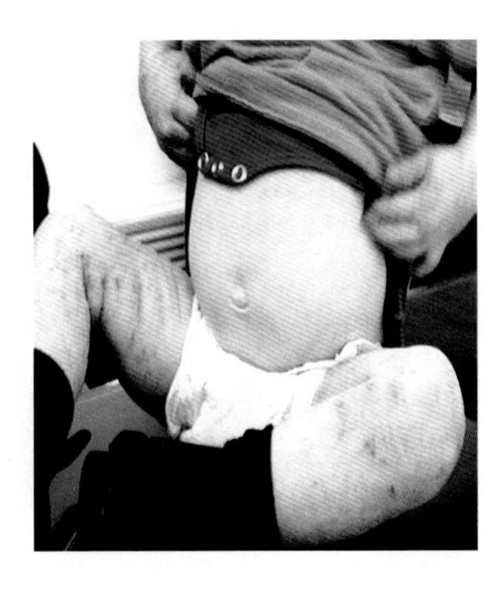

Fig. 1 Itch in eczema. The most troublesome symptom in eczema is the constant itch, affecting normal daily activities (school activities), temperament and sleep of the child.

The prevalence of AD is the highest in infancy, and the natural course in most is remission during childhood. In Singapore, AD affects more than 20% of young children below the age of two. Worldwide, there has been an increase in the prevalence of AD during the last 30 years (cfr. The ISAAC studies), which is in parallel with the increase of prevalence of atopy. In older children, the prevalence of AD is lower, usually between 10-15% of children. In most children, AD starts during infancy, but AD can also start at an older age, even during adulthood. Usually, AD gets better when the child gets older, but many children with AD have persistent lesions during many years, up till puberty. The major symptom of AD is **ITCH** (Fig. 1), which affects the quality of life considerably, causing sleep disturbances and learning difficulties.

AD is a very troublesome disease, mainly because of its stigmatizing effect, especially when the AD lesions are localized in the face: children with AD will isolate themselves (i.e. not wanting to come out of their rooms, pretending they are sick on school days), inducing a lot of psychological and social problems in children.

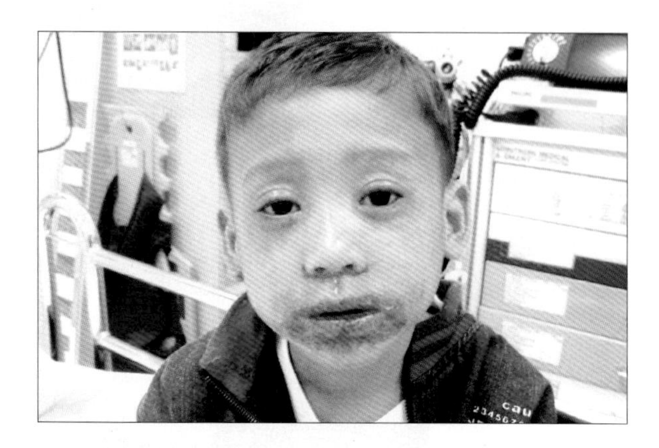

Fig. 2 Severe eczema in the face leading to social isolation of the child.

1. Pruritus
2. Typical form and distribution of skin lesions
3. Chronic or recurrent dermatitis
4. A personal or family history of atopy

Fig. 3 4 major criteria of AD.

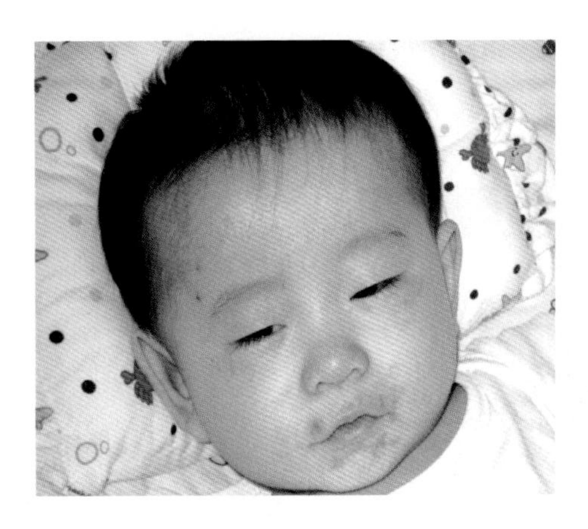

Fig. 4 Mild eczema around mouth in baby. Mild eczema in around the mouth of a cute 8 months old baby. This type of eczema is usually non-allergic and caused by hypersensitivity of the skin to the child's own saliva. Usually mild treatment (moisturizing) will be able to control the lesions and most babies grow out of this type of eczema.

Symptoms of AD

AD has no specific skin signs and comprises a number of atypical dermatological characteristics such as ichtyosis (dry skin), erythema (redness), excoriation (interruption of the skin), scratching lesions, lichenification (thickening of the skin), infected lesions (blisters, pus formation), and hypopigmentation or hyperpigmentation in old lesions (see Fig. 2). The diagnosis of AD is usually based on clinical assessment and on established criteria, such as the criteria of Hanifin and Rajka. (Fig. 3)

Except for dry skin, children do not have symptoms from birth (see Fig. 4). The first symptoms of AD usually appear before the age of three months. The exact triggers of the first lesions of AD are unknown. Usually, allergic reactions are not present at that early age. In 80% of children with AD, the lesions appear before the age of one, and in 90% before the age of five. The most invariable symptom is ITCH (= **pruritus),** which can sometimes be very intense and cause severe sleep disturbances (insomnia). The

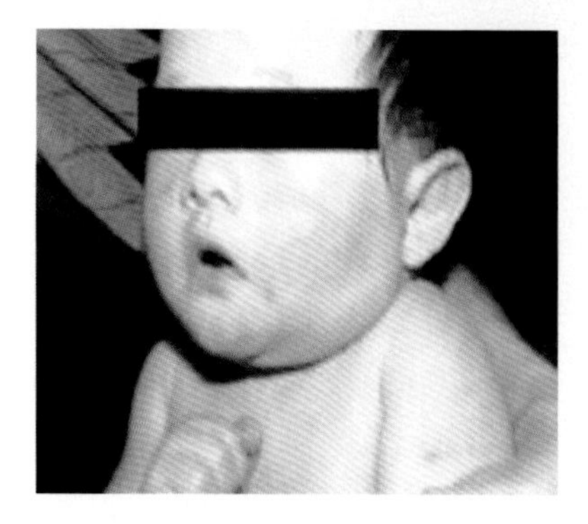
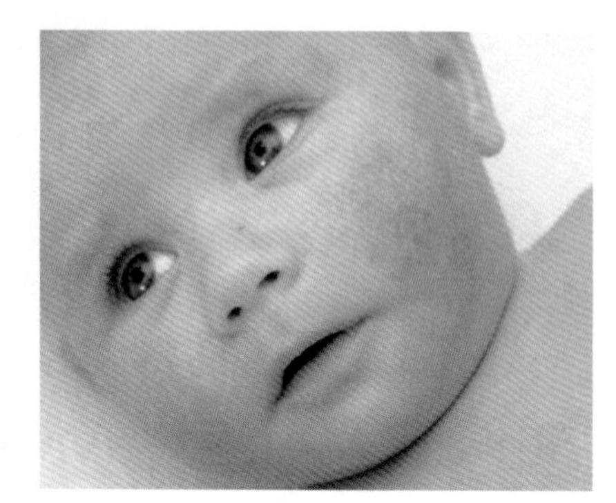

Fig. 5 Severe eczema in face of 2 infants. Infants with severe eczema in the face, due to an underlying allergy to cow's milk. The lesions on the cheeks are very crusty, suggesting secondary infection.

distribution profile of the disease varies with age and is characterized by the predominance of certain skin lesions:

Infants

The area's most commonly affected are the face (see Fig. 5), scalp, neck, arms and legs (especially the front of the knees and the back of the elbows), and trunk. The rash usually does not appear in the diaper area. The rash presents itself most commonly as dry, red, scaling areas on the baby's cheeks. The rash is often crusted or oozes fluid and rubbing and scratching can lead to frequent infections.

Older children (age two to 11 years)

The symptoms may appear for the first time or may be a continuation of the infant phase. The rash occurs primarily on the back of the legs and arms, on the neck, and in areas that bend, such as the back of the knees and the inside of the elbows (Fig. 6). Wrists and ankles are also commonly involved. The rash is usually dry (Fig. 7). But it may go through

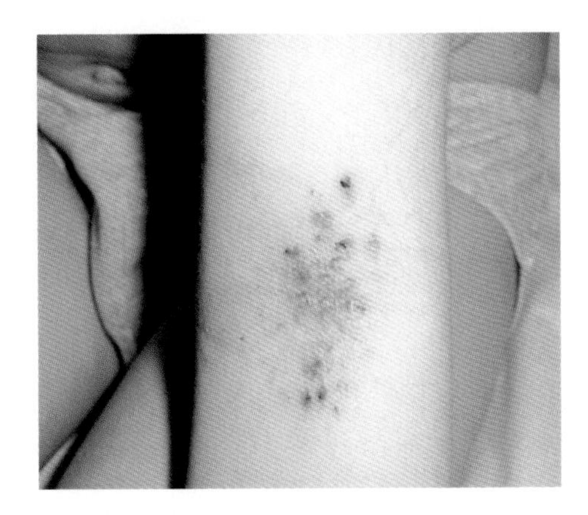

Fig. 6 Elbow eczema in a 5-year old child. Eczema in elbow fold of a 5-year old boy who is allergic to house dust mites.

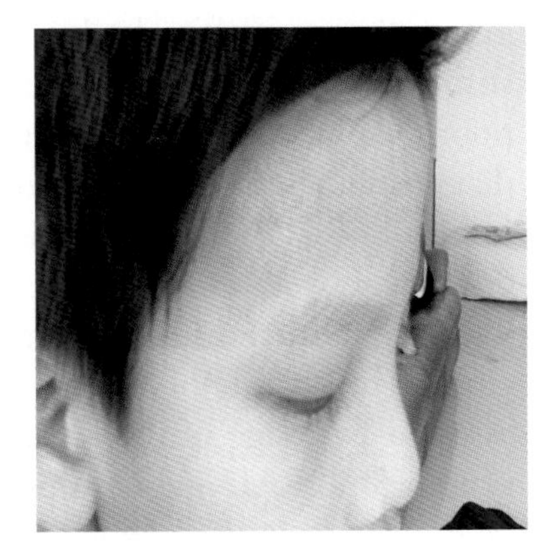

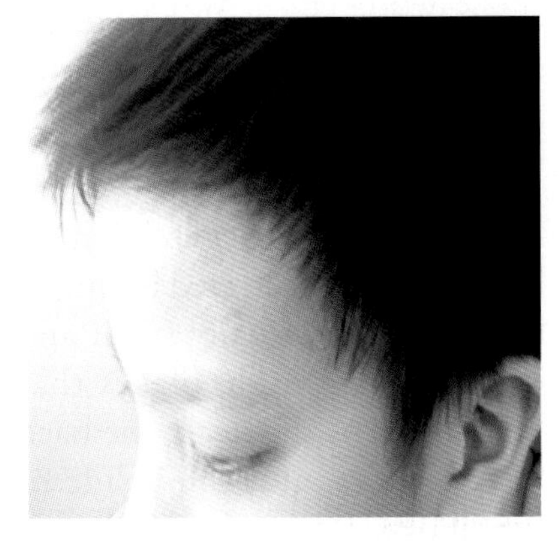

Fig. 7 Eczema on the forehead in an 8-year-old boy who is very allergic to house dust mites.

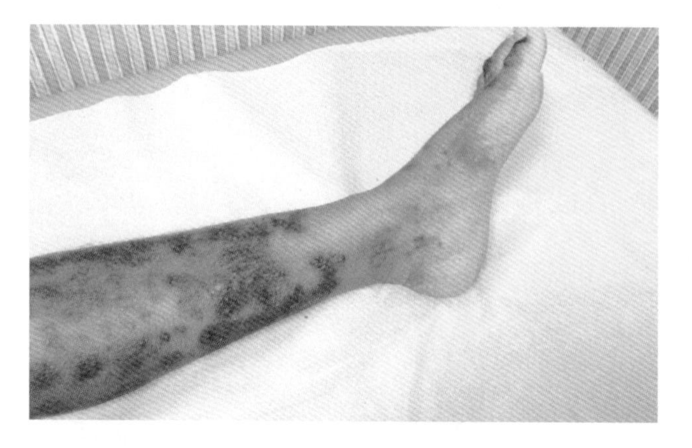

Fig. 8 Old hyperpigmented lesions. Severe chronic *infected* eczema in an adolescent. The lesions are hyperpigmented and infected. The hyperpigmentation is a consequence of the eczema, and can last for a lifetime.

stages from an acute oozing rash to a red, dry subacute rash, and to a chronic rash that causes the skin to thicken (lichenification). Lichenification often occurs after the rash goes away. Rubbing and scratching can lead to infections.

Adolescents and adults

AD often improves as children get older. The areas affected by atopic dermatitis are usually small and commonly include places that bend, such as the neck, the back of the knees, and the inside of the elbows. Rashes can also affect the face, wrists, and forearms. Rashes are rare in the groin area. Usually the skin remains very dry, with hyperlinearity of hands and feet, and with pronounced lichenification (Fig. 8).

The diagnosis of AD is generally not difficult, but in some cases the symptoms are poorly defined. In this event, the diagnostic criteria of Hanifin and Lobitz (or Rajka) are useful. These criteria are well known and used by many clinicians all over the globe. The severity of AD can be assessed by usage of the scoring system SCORAD, which might be important in the follow-up of the disease or in standardization of criteria of severity as needed in

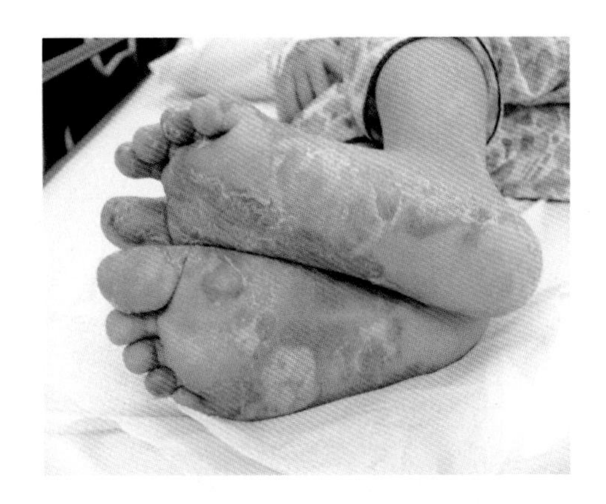

Fig. 9 Infected eczema of feet. Severe infection of the feet in a child with eczema. The infection is caused by *Staphylococcus aureus*, and was a result of undertreatment of the lesions.

clinical trials. The clinical course is characterized by variability and unpredictability. The asymptomatic intervals usually become extended as the child ages. It is estimated that in 60% of children with severe AD requiring hospitalization, symptoms will persist above the age of 20. In 95% of milder cases, symptoms disappear before the age of 20.

Complications of AD

AD, especially severe AD or non-treated AD, may lead to the development of a number of complications, which might have considerable impact on the quality of life of children. Complications of AD include: cutaneous infections (especially with *Staphylococcus aureus*), common warts and molluscum contagiosum, ocular complications, contact dermatitis (to creams containing corticosteroids or antibiotics), and sleep disturbances inducing learning difficulties.

Infections of the skin (Figs. 9-11)

AD lesions are usually open lesions, because the skin is

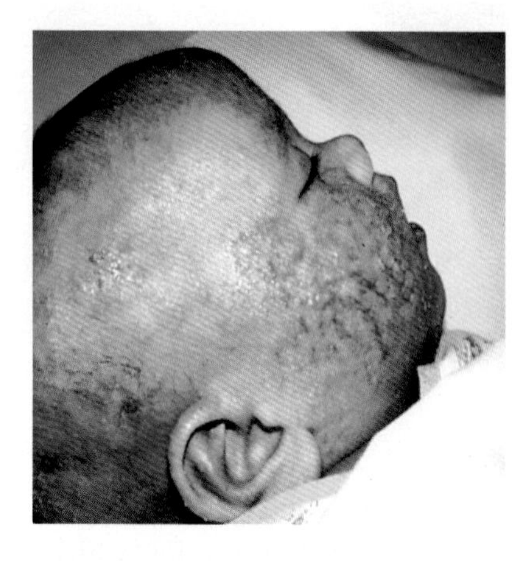

Fig. 10 Baby with infected eczema of face.

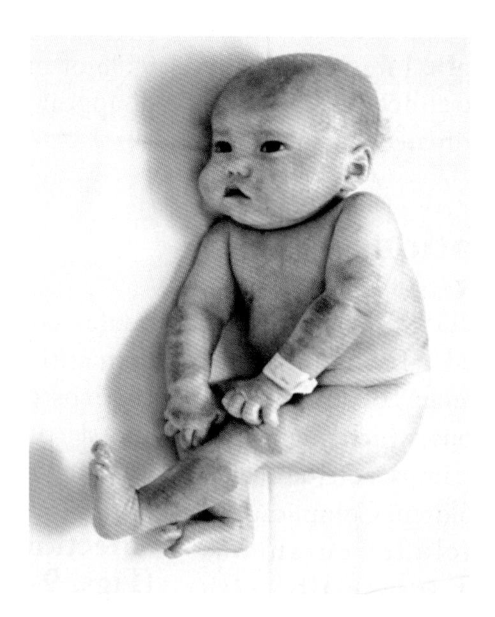

Fig. 11 Baby with severe infected generalized eczema.

interrupted by the continuous scratching of the child. Children with AD scratch all the time, even during their sleep. Therefore, infection and colonization with bacteria of AD lesions, even of the so-called normal skin in-between the lesions, with bacteria is very common. Almost all children with AD have a colonized skin from an early age on. The most common bacteria found on the skin of AD children are *Staphylococcus aureus*. It has been known that this type of bacterium has an exceptional preference for colonizing AD lesions. Furthermore, the bacterium is able **to infect** the lesions, causing pus formation, and fever in cases of severe infection.

The cause of the increased susceptibility of patients with AD to *Staphylococcus aureus* colonization lies in the inability of skin cells (keratinocytes) to secrete antimicrobial peptides, which suppress bacterial colonization. On the other hand, colonization with *Staphylococcus aureus* will induce persistence and worsening of AD, without signs of infection. Proteins of the bacterium on itself can maintain the skin inflammation by acting as allergens, and by inducing cell activation in the skin. Therefore, these proteins are also called "super antigens". Once the skin has become colonized with *Staphylococcus aureus*, treatment becomes more difficult, as most of the anti-inflammatory creams, such as corticosteroids, will become less effective. Other mechanisms by which *Staphylococcus aureus* can worsen AD are induction of specific IgE against the bacterium, and secretion of enzymes (proteases) that can destruct the skin barrier. ***Therefore, keeping the concentration of bacteria on the skin low is one of the main approaches in the treatment of AD.***

Apart from bacterial infections, a number of viruses can induce infection of the skin in AD patients. One of the most severe complications is **eczema herpeticum** (Fig. 12), which is a severe, disseminated herpes infection of AD, caused by herpes simplex virus (type 1 and 2). Eczema herpeticum results in a severe disseminated infection, involving multiple organs, such as the eyes, brain, lung, liver and others, and can be fatal. Treatment with systemic antiviral drugs, such as acyclovir or valaciclovir, is therefore needed.

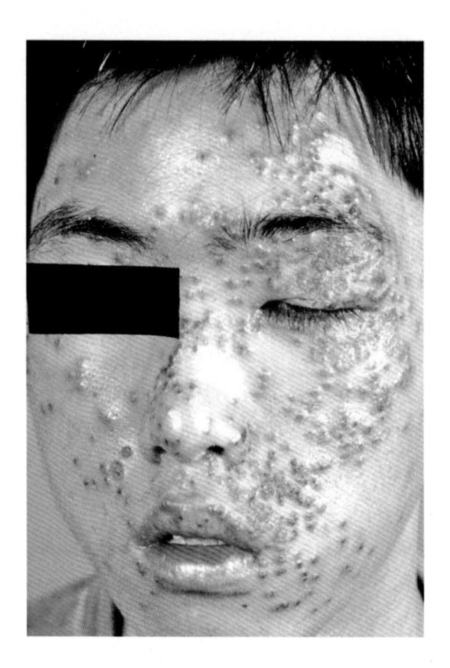

Fig. 12 Eczema herpeticum (courtesy of the National Skin Centre, Singapore).

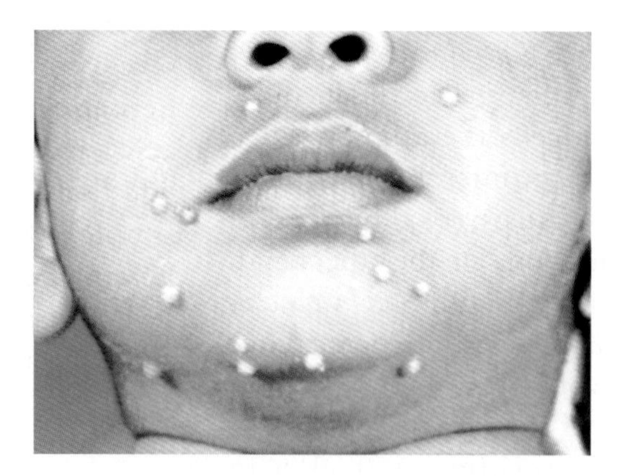

Fig. 13 Molluscum contagiosum (a viral infection causing a specific type of warts) is a frequent complication of eczema (courtesy of the National Skin Centre, Singapore).

When smallpox vaccination was still being routinely administered, the vaccinia virus used in the smallpox vaccine could cause a similar syndrome if the patient had active eczema. This condition was called *eczema vaccinatum*. Eczema herpeticum and eczema vaccinatum are collectively known as **Kaposi's varicelliform eruption**. Smallpox vaccination is contraindicated in patients with AD unless there is imminent danger of exposure to smallpox.

Other viral infections of the skin in children with AD can cause common warts or molluscum contagiosum (Fig. 13). If severe, these lesions sometimes need to be removed surgically.

Psychological problems in children with AD

Itch is the most troublesome symptom in all children with AD, affecting their sleep and their ability to concentrate in school. Sleep disturbances of children with AD include: difficulty falling asleep, diminished total sleep, frequent awakenings, difficult awakenings, daytime tiredness, and irritability. A large number of studies have been performed on the quality of life in children with eczema. Moreover, from clinical practice, it is clear that AD can cause a lot of misery, not only to the child, but affecting the whole family.

Examples mentioned by parents on their child with AD:

1. On the child's physical health
   "He scratches throughout the night... his sheets are bloody... disfiguring himself..."
2. On the child's emotional health
   "He is a crying uncomfortable child... is miserable..."
3. On the child's physical functioning
   "I won't let him play in the backyard, sandboxes, or swim..."
4. On the child's social functioning
   "If you don't stop scratching, no one is going to want to play with you..."

All children with AD should be treated optimally. This will avoid complications such as skin infections, and major psychological problems for child and family!

Especially in cases of severe AD, the disease can be extremely disabling, causing overwhelming psychological problems in child and parents. Many studies have shown the burden of AD on child and family, reporting its social, emotional, and financial impact. Children with AD have a lower health-related quality of life and greater psychological distress than healthy children. Children with AD often have behavioral problems such as increased dependency, fearfulness and sleep difficulties, resulting in impaired school results, isolation, and depression. Studies have shown that families with a child affected by AD had a lower quality of life than families of healthy children. Parents describe a general burden of extra care and psychological pressure, including feelings of guilt, exhaustion, frustration, resentment, and helplessness.

Is AD an allergic disease?

A large number of children with AD have other signs of other allergic diseases, such as asthma, rhinitis, or food allergy. Usually, the respiratory symptoms begin later than the skin symptoms and many clinicians have noted the peculiar and unexplained tendency for AD and asthma to alternate in their courses. This phenomenon is not constant, however, as both can flare simultaneously. Moreover, about 30% of all children with AD will develop asthma, and when considering severe AD the prevalence is even higher (60-80%), depending on the results of different studies.

Switching from AD to asthma and, subsequently, rhinitis is also called The Allergic March. The underlying mechanisms of switching from AD to asthma or rhinitis are unknown, but might be related to specific organ sensitivity to an allergy and to the type of allergen to which allergic reactions develop.

The highest levels of IgE have been detected in patients suffering from both AD and asthma. It is not yet known whether there is a real causal relationship between these high levels and AD, or whether this is just an expression of the atopic constitution. In some patients, however, IgE might be important in the pathogenesis of AD, while in others it is not.

Nowadays there is still a lot of debate ongoing on the exact role of allergic reactions in AD.

The following observations have been made:

1. Increased total serum IgE has been recorded in about 80% of patients (less in infants). In addition, there is a correlation between total serum IgE and severity of AD (also in infants).
2. Positive skin prick tests and positive specific IgE to a number of inhaled allergens, especially house dust mites, and food allergens are found in the majority of patients with moderate to severe eczema.
3. Positive family antecedents of atopic diseases are found in the majority of patients.
4. Of subjects with AD, 50%-80% suffer also from asthma and/or rhino-conjunctivitis.

A positive skin prick test to an allergen still does not mean the AD lesions are triggered by this particular allergen. The prick test (or the determination of specific IgE in the blood) is known to yield false positive and false negative results. A possible explanation for the false negative results is that the skin lesions are induced by non-IgE-dependent mechanisms. On the other hand, a positive prick test corresponds to a clinically detectable allergy (by a provocation test) **in only about 25% of AD patients.** Moreover, in young children, prick tests are more frequently negative than in older children.

As AD is often associated with allergic reactions, it does not prove that the AD lesions are caused by the underlying allergy.

Therefore, different situations are possible:

1. In a number of children food allergens will induce reactions, such as urticaria (hives) on top of the AD lesions, inducing an indirect worsening of the AD.
2. In a number of children the underlying allergy is not involved in the AD lesions (i.e. independent findings).
3. In a number of children the allergy is a consequence of the AD, and is caused because the eczematous skin allows allergens to easily penetrate the body (see also skin barrier defects). The allergy can than become involved into the maintaining of the AD lesions.

To prove whether or not an allergy is really involved in AD, the only valuable test is a provocation test: give the allergen (usual food) to the child and see what happens. There are strict scientific criteria for provocation tests. The best design is the double-blind placebo-controlled test. In this test neither the investigator nor the patient knows what allergen is administrated and results are compared to those of a placebo administration, mainly to exclude the role of possible underlying psychological factors.

Provocation testing with allergens should always be performed in a hospital (never at home), as severe reactions can occur. Therefore, the need of a provocation test should be judged against its therapeutic consequences, and against the possible risks that can occur.

Double-blind placebo-controlled provocation tests = golden standard

The history of the child with AD usually contains insufficient information to establish a clear link between exposure to an allergen (food) and the appearance of AD lesions. Parents often report their child to be "allergic" to a particular food, but when a provocation test is carried out, this food seldom seems to have any effect on the skin lesions. The opposite is often equally true: clearly positive provocation results are obtained by foods that the parents did not suspect. In a large number of studies the value of double-blind placebo-controlled provocation tests (DBPCPT) was demonstrated.

Taking together the results from different studies, it has been shown that food allergy can play a role in AD. Most positive reactions to food occur in young children with severe types of AD. However, only a limited number of foods are involved in AD. These include: eggs, cow's milk, soy, and wheat.

Three examples:

1. In children with severe AD, challenged by Sampson and McCaskill, 63 children out of 113 (56%) showed positive reactions to food, using the DBPCPT. Cow's milk, eggs, and peanuts were responsible for 72% of the positive DBPCPT.
2. In another study, on 25 children with severe AD, we could demonstrate, by DBPCPT, that foods are able to induce exacerbations of AD in 24 out of 25 of the subjects. In that same study it was also found that food additives, tyramine and acetylsalicylic acid, were able to cause exacerbations of AD.
3. In children with mild to moderate AD, the role of foods seems to be less important. In a study by Burks on 165 children with mild to moderate AD, it was found that 60% of the patients had positive skin prick tests to food and only 39% showed positive DBPCPT. Moreover, most positive reactions were found in the younger age group.

The role of food allergy is greater in infants compared to adults whose AD is rarely influenced by dietary factors (Table 1). The prevalence of food allergy in infants with AD has been estimated at up to 40%. However, prevalence of food allergy is very much dependent on the severity of AD. In infants with severe AD, food allergy can be involved in more than 70% of them.

Table 1 Most Common Food Allergies in Children with Eczema

Infants	Preschooolers	Older Children
- cow's milk - eggs - wheat - soy	- cow's milk - eggs - peanut - tree-nuts - fish - shellfish - sesame - fruits	- peanut - tree-nuts - fish - shellfish - sesame - fruits - bird's nest

House dust mites and AD: a causal relationship?

In a great number of older children with AD (not in infants), positive reactions (skin prick test and specific IgE) to a number of inhaled allergens can be found, especially to house dust mites. The exact roles of these allergic reactions in AD are still a matter of debate and are not accepted as involved in AD by every researcher. For some, they are merely a manifestation of the atopic constitution.

There is, however, evidence that these allergic reactions to inhaled allergens, such as house dust mites, can be triggers of AD lesions:

1. After provocation studies with house dust mites AD lesions may occur. This was shown in a number of well-controlled studies in the lab.
2. In other studies it was shown that AD improved by cleaning the patient's bedrooms, especially in children (results were not convincing in adults).
3. In the blood of patients with AD, specific lymphocytes were detected that start proliferating after contact of their blood with HDM, suggesting that HDM can induce inflammation in these patients.
4. When house dust mites are applied on the skin of AD patients by patch test, new AD lesions can be induced. These skin reactions, which are delayed in time (positive after 24 – 72 hours), did not occur in allergic asthma and allergic rhinitis, and, therefore,

Table 2 Different Triggers for AD in Children 4

- Food allergens
- Inhalant allergens
- Contact allergens
- Bacterial colonization of the skin
- Irritant substances (soap, wool, perspiration, hot water, etc)
- Cold climate
- Psychological factors (stress)
- Infections (fever)

seemed to be specific for AD. Microscopy of the patch test reactions shows many similarities to the clinically involved skin in AD.

These different types of evidence suggest that the elimination of house dust mites should be advised in a number of patients with AD. The role of other inhaled allergens (pets, pollen) is less clear, but some anecdotic stories (such as: more AD after playing with a cat, or after playing on the grass) suggest their involvement.

Conclusions: is AD an allergic disease?

AD is a complex disease in which a great number of environmental factors are involved, including food allergens and inhalant allergens, but also non-allergic triggers (Table 2). In young children with severe AD, food allergens, such as cow's milk and hen's eggs, should be considered as triggering factors. In older children, however, the role of food seems to be less important. In these patients, inhaled allergens, such as house dust mites, might maintain the chronic lesions.

The skin barrier defects in AD

AD has a strong familial predisposition. Screening in families with AD has implicated genetic abnormalities that are associated with skin barrier quality and with abnormalities of the immune system (i.e. allergic genotype). Therefore,

At the start of AD, usually during the first three months of life, most infants show no allergic reactions. Therefore, it could be that allergy is a consequence of the abnormal skin barrier, allowing allergens to penetrate more easily in the bodies, and triggering the immune system. After allergic sensitization, allergens take over and become triggers of AD.

since recently, clinical research has focused more on the abnormalities of the skin of children with AD, suggesting that AD mainly occurs in children who are born with **a "bad quality" of the skin.** These studies are difficult to perform, mainly because they need the availability of skin biopsies (pieces of skin to study under the microscope), which are very difficult to obtain for ethical reasons. Therefore, this type of research was mainly performed on adult volunteers, and only limited information is available of the skin features of newborns or young children with AD. However, from the limited research that is available, it was shown that the skin of children who have AD have specific features (such as increased dryness, increased water loss through the skin, and increased pH) that lead to an inferior functioning of the skin, also referred to as an **impaired skin barrier function**. Certain biochemical abnormalities, which all have a specific genetic constitution, have been associated with an inferior skin barrier: such as decreased expression of certain proteins in the skin that maintain an optimal skin barrier (example: decreased expression of **filaggrin, cornulin and loricin**) or increased expression of certain enzymes that might decrease the tightness of the skin cells (example: increased production in the skin of chymotrypsin). All these abnormalities make the skin become very dry and sensitive to the environment, which increases the risk of developing AD.

The exact mechanisms of the start of AD (initiation) in a newborn baby with a decreased skin barrier are unknown, and the exact causes of the beginning of the inflammation in the skin, leading to AD, have yet to be identified. Three related observations have been witnessed:

1. At the start of AD in young children, allergic reactions are not present or detectable in most of the children.
2. In some children with AD, auto-antibodies against skin cells (such as keratinocytes) can be found. The origin or role of these antibodies are unknown, but it has not been excluded that these auto-antibodies might initiate AD in newborns. These auto-antibodies might induce skin inflammation and be at the origin of AD.
3. Young children with dry skin are very itchy. The initiation of AD could be a consequence of mechanical triggering (rubbing, scratching).

During the last 30 years an increase of skin barrier defects has been noted in children, in parallel with the increase of AD. A major cause of this is the increased use of water and soap to wash the skin. In a study from the UK it was shown that the usage of water for personal washing has increased from 11 liters/day (period 1960–1981) to 51 liters/day (period 1995–2001). Therefore, it could be that the increase of AD during the last 30 years is due to an increase of allergy plus an increase of the prevalence of skin barrier defects.

Based on current knowledge of skin barrier defects, the role of allergy and the role of staphylococcal infections, a hypothetical model of AD can be constructed, associating the underlying causes of AD with the chronic inflammation. From this model it seems that the underlying triggers of AD differ with age. **Treatment should therefore be adapted according to the triggers and age of the child.**

The hypothetical model of AD in children constitutes three phases, according to age (see Fig. 14).

AD in early infancy

AD starts with a defective skin barrier (genetically determined). The first lesions of inflammation are due to scratching or rubbing.

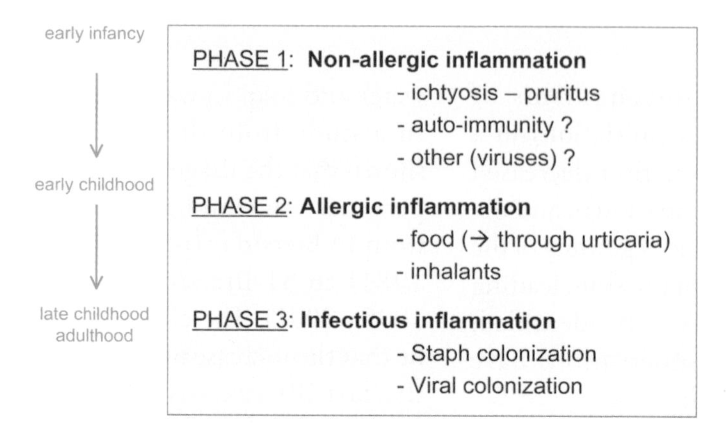

Fig. 14 Hypothetic model of AD: the 3 phases of eczema in children.

Allergic reactions are not present, and the role of auto-antibodies or other triggers (environmental factors, such as viruses) still needs to be elucidated.

AD in early childhood (infants, preschoolers)

Allergic reactions (mainly foods) can appear, as a consequence of the defective skin barrier, if the child has an underlying allergic constitution. If not, the AD persists without allergy being involved, and is maintained by mechanical and other (non-identified) non-allergic triggers.

AD in older children and adults

In older children, chronic colonization of the skin by *Staphylococcus aureus* becomes an important maintenance factor of AD. In the meantime, allergic reactions to inhalant allergens become more prominent, especially allergic reactions to the different house dust mites. The AD becomes a chronic inflammation maintained by Staphylococcus aureus colonization (of which the proteins act as super-antigens that maintain inflammation) and by house dust mites. The role of food allergy has decreased, and older children with AD have no underlying food allergy. If there is a food allergy, this allergy will mainly induce urticaria (hives) and angioedema (swelling), having only an indirect effect on AD lesions.

Based on current knowledge on allergy and skin barrier defects, it has become obvious that AD is a very complex disease and that a large number of specific features may be involved in the underlying mechanisms of AD. In some children it will be mainly the skin barriers defects that cause the AD, while in others it will be mainly allergic reactions (and a minimal skin barrier defect) or the auto-antibodies against the skin proteins. Therefore, AD should be considered **as a SYNDROME** (i.e. the atopic eczema/dermatitis syndrome or AEDS), made up by different subtypes, and treatment should be individualized, according to the subtype of AD.

Treatment of AD

Treatment in AD (Table 3) should be individualized according to the age of the child and according to the type and severity of AD. In some cases of severe infected AD, hospitalization might be necessary for intravenous treatment with corticosteroids and/or antibiotics.

GENERAL RULES ARE:

1. Moisturize, moisturize, and moisturize …

Nowadays more attention is paid to the type of moisturizer that is used, as it seems that not all moisturizers give similar effects. Moisturizing is now focused on restoring the skin barrier, by applying creams of which the composition mimics the skin barrier (i.e. moisturizers that result in barrier repair or pathogenesis-based-therapy), directed at the lipid biochemical abnormalities that underlie the barrier defect in AD.

Therefore, moisturizers containing lipid replacements (such as ceramides and free fatty acids) seem to be more effective, especially in young children.

Table 3 Focus of the Treatment of AD, According to Age Group

INFANTS	... on MOISTURIZING
PRESCHOOLERS	... on ALLERGY
OLDER CHILDREN	... on AVOIDANCE OF BACTERIAL COLONIZATION

2. **Keep the skin clean and free of bacterial colonization by using mild local antiseptics, such as chlorhexidin. Avoid the usage of antibiotics, except in severe skin infection. Repeated usage of antibiotics will result in an increased resistance of the bacteria, causing the AD to become more difficult to control.**
3. **Use mild and safe corticosteroids, but only on patches of AD and not on dry skin. Be restrictive with corticosteroids in the face, and replace them with pimecrolimus or tacrolimus.**
4. **Oral antihistamines have only a limited effect on itch and it is mainly the old and sedating antihistamines that show mild effectiveness, such as hydroxizin and ketotifen. The new antihistamines (such as cetirizine, levocetirizine, loratadine and desloratidine) have no effect on itch in AD.**
5. **AD is complex, and, therefore, the treatment of AD should be tailored and offered as "a whole package" of medications and interventions.**

A. In infants

- Usually AD starts with a dry itchy skin during the first months of life. Therefore, treatment should be focused on **moisturizing** the skin, using moisturizers that restore the skin barrier.
- Furthermore, the colonization by bacteria should be avoided. This can be done by using mild local antiseptics or soaps containing antiseptics. It is

important to mention that after contact of the skin with water, moisturizing should be performed.

- Mild lesions of AD can be safely treated with mild local corticosteroids, such as hydrocortisone 1% creams. It is advisable to avoid corticosteroids in the face (at all ages), because of the possibility that long-term usage of corticosteroids in the face will induce mild thinning of the skin, although this is extremely rare. Therefore, to treat AD patches in the face it is advised to use creams containing pimecrolimus, which is a non-steroidal anti-inflammatory medicine, blocking the activation of lymphocytes. In older children, tacrolimus creams can also be used.
- Usage of oral antihistamines to treat itch is not advisable for infants, except in exceptional cases. Usage of low doses of ketotifen seems to be preferential for these infants.

B. Young children (preschoolers)

- The same treatment is applicable as for infants: moisturizing, antiseptics, mild corticosteroids, and pimecrolimus (or tacrolimus) in the face.
- In the case of an underlying proven food allergy, the food should be avoided as much as possible. Contacts with food can also occur through smelling. It has been shown that dust of kitchens contains traces of antigens from milk and eggs. Therefore, in cases of severe food allergy it is advisable to abandon the food from the home of the child.
- Regular swimming in a swimming pool containing chlorine is advisable to keep colonization with bacteria low. However, the water will dry the skin, and, therefore, extensive moisturizing after swimming is advisable. Furthermore, swimming should be restricted to 10-15 minutes, to avoid extreme drying of the skin. In cases where active AD lesions are present, avoiding the sun is advised.

C. Older children

- The same treatment is applicable as for younger children and infants: moisturizing, antiseptics,

id corticosteroids, and pimecrolimus (or tacrolimus) in the face.
- In cases of house dust mite allergy, avoidance of dust is advisable, especially in the bedroom (clean mattress and pillow).
- Treatment should be focused on reducing skin colonization by bacteria. Regular swimming in a swimming pool containing chlorine in the water and usage of antiseptics is essential for older children with AD. Local antibiotics can be used in cases of infectious flare up of AD lesions.

Other treatments in AD

1. Usage of probiotics, prebiotics, and synbiotics

Bacterial products, such as probiotics, prebiotics (= sugars to increase the body's own bacterial flora) and synbiotics (= a combination of probiotics and prebiotics) have no major role in the treatment of established AD, as only a few studies reported mild improvement of AD after administration of bacterial products. In contrast, it seems that there is a role for bacterial products in the prevention of AD, although not all studies showed positive results. From the limited information we have now, bacterial products are able to prevent AD if they are started during pregnancy, and if they are given in combination with breastfeeding. Studies from Australia and Singapore on formula milks containing probiotics were unable to show any effect of the intervention. More studies are underway, and for the moment the data is conflicting and confusing. Therefore, it is felt that we should wait for the results of the new studies before making firm conclusions.

2. Treatment of severe exacerbations of AD

In some children with severe AD, severe exacerbations of the skin lesions (such as severe infection) might need hospitalization for systemic treatment. These children are than treated with intravenous antibiotics and/or corticosteroids. Regular preventive treatment is a way to avoid hospitalization, (also called proactive treatment) and all children with AD should be encouraged to use their treatment (especially moisturizers and antiseptics) on a daily basis. In some children it might be necessary to use stronger treatments that suppress the ongoing inflammation in the skin, such as azathioprine or cyclosporine. The role of immunotherapy (such as SLIT) needs further study, but the first results of the usage of SLIT in children with mild to moderate AD seems promising.

Prognosis of AD

In most children the prognosis of AD is favorable, as most of them will grow out of their skin problems. However, about one in three children with AD will develop respiratory allergy (asthma or rhinitis) later in life. Usually, AD gets better when the child gets older, but many children with severe AD have persistent lesions during many years, and in some the lesions will persist during adulthood. In most cases, there is a decrease in flare-ups of acute exacerbations, and the symptomfree intervals get longer, although the dryness of the skin remains. It has been shown in follow-up studies that 60% of children with severe AD will still have symptoms at the age of 20. In more than 90% of children with mild to moderate AD, symptoms disappear before the age of 20. Most adults who suffered from AD during childhood will still have a persistence of dry and itchy skin. Moreover, undertreated AD can lead to the persistence of severe rest lesions (scaring of the skin). The rest lesions of AD are usually hyperpigmented lesions (Fig. 15) for which there is no treatment.

Risk factors for a poor prognosis of AD are:

1. **Severe AD: the more severe, the worse the prognosis**
2. **Early allergic sensitization: the more allergic reactions involved, the worse the prognosis**

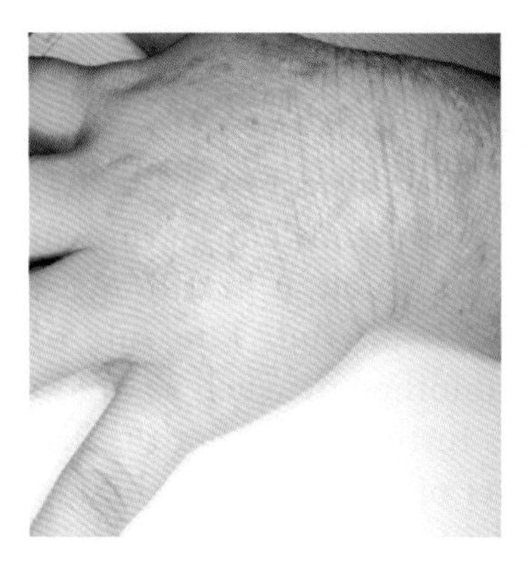

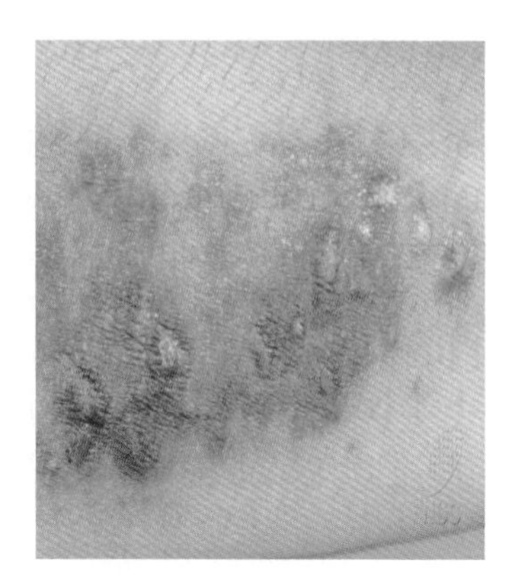

Fig. 15 Dry skin with lichenification and hyperpigmented lesions. Most children grow out of their eczema; however, the dry skin with the lichenification (hyperlinearity of the skin) or hyperpigmentation remains.

Other types of eczema in children

a. Seborrhoeic eczema

This type of eczema appears in infants, usually between two weeks to two months of life as red, scaly rashes on the trunk (back) and scalp. The lesions are red and crusty, and there can be a yellowish scaly crust on the scalp (known as cradle cap). Sometimes, distinguishing from early AD is difficult, even impossible. However, this type of eczema has a better prognosis, as most infants will recover very quickly, as a consequence of a local treatment. The underlying mechanisms of seborrhoeic eczema are fairly unknown. For some researchers, this type of eczema has the same underlying mechanisms as AD, and is also closely linked with an underlying atopic constitution. The main treatments for infants are **emollient creams**, but mild

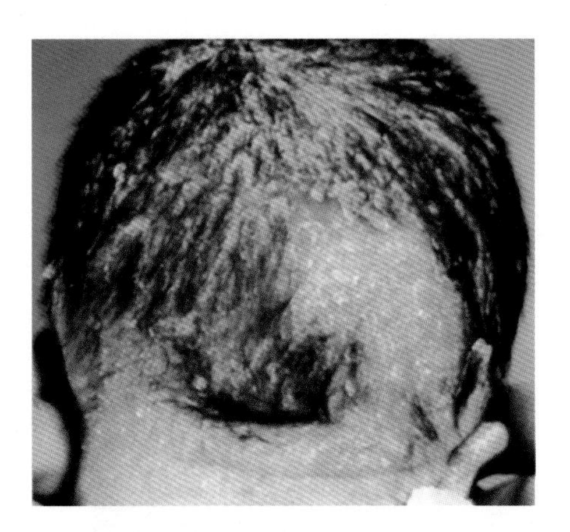

Fig. 16 Seborrhoeic eczema (courtesy of the National Skin Centre, Singapore).

corticosteroid creams may be needed. Cradle cap, which is a manifestation of seborrhoeic eczema (Fig. 16), can be loosened with a mixture of salicylic acid in aqueous cream, which is then washed out with baby shampoo. Oils such as olive oil are also long-standing remedies for de-scaling cradle cap. Seborrhoeic eczema can also occur in older children and during adulthood, although it is not sure whether the underlying mechanisms are similar to those in infants.

b. Contact eczema or contact dermatitis

Contact eczema (Fig. 17) is a localized rash or irritation of the skin caused by an inflammation of the skin, as a result of direct contact of the skin with a foreign substance. IgE is not involved in contact dermatitis, as this is a delayed type of immune response in which T-cells are activated. Substances that cause contact dermatitis in many people include "poisonous" plants such as poison ivy, some metals (nickel, such as in jewels or piercings), cleaning solutions, detergents, cosmetics, perfumes, leather (shoes), and industrial chemicals. Avoidance of the substance is the most effective treatment. Local application of corticosteroids reduces the inflammation.

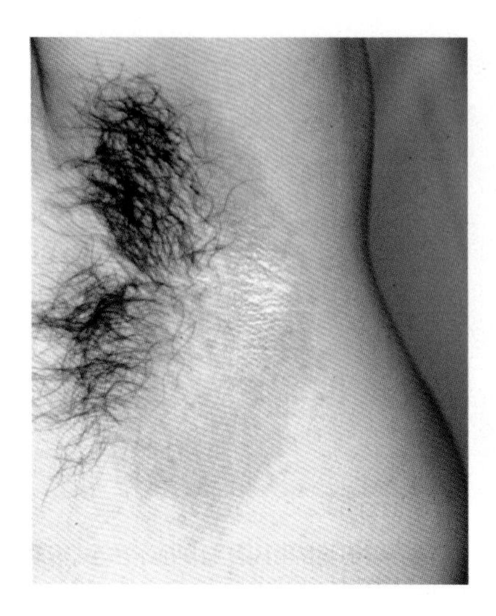

Fig. 17 Contact eczema. Contact eczema in a boy to a deodorant spray (courtesy of the National Skin Centre, Singapore).

Furthermore, all these type of eczema should be distinguished from other diseases. The most common diseases from which AD should be distinguished are scabies (Fig. 18) and psoriasis (Fig. 19).

General conclusion

AD is a complex disease of which many aspects are yet not understood. The role of allergy is still uncertain, as a large number of patients (especially young children) show no evidence of an underlying allergic constitution. Recently, more attention was given to the role of a defective skin barrier. Currently, it seems that many "players" are involved in AD, including the skin barrier defects, allergic reactions, and chronic colonization with *Staphylococcus aureus*. A number of exacerbating factors are still largely unknown. AD is the result of this complex interplay between the different exacerbating factors, which can differ in time and which are different from patient to patient.

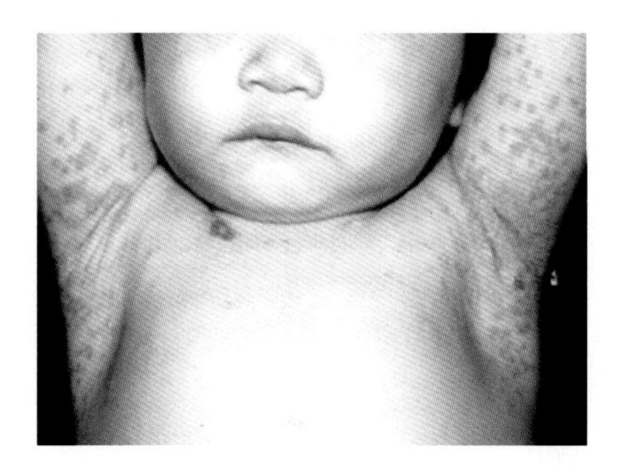

Fig. 18 Scabies can resemble eczema (courtesy of the National Skin Centre, Singapore).

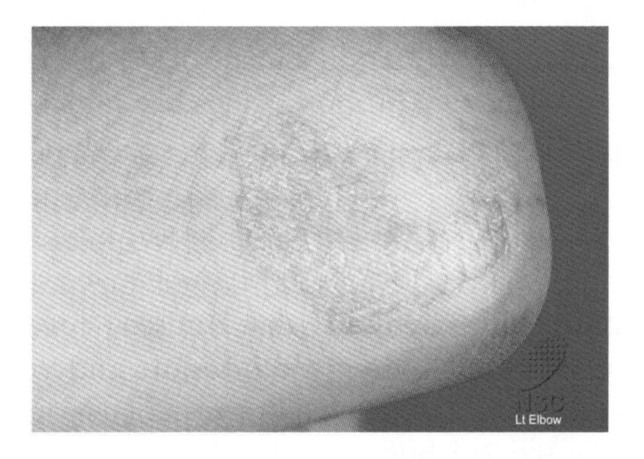

Fig. 19 Psoriasis. In some children psoriasis (which is an uncommon disease in children) can look very similar to eczema. The picture is of psoriasis at a boy's elbow (courtesy of the National Skin Centre, Singapore).

7

Urticaria and Angioedema

What is urticaria – angioedema?

Urticaria of hives is an itchy rash that is raised ("hives"), and consists of wheals with pale interiors and well-defined red margins. Hives can be irregular, big or small, rounded or flat-topped, but are always elevated above the surrounding skin. Urticaria is usually well circumscribed but may be coalescent and will blanch with pressure. The hives typically last less than four hours but they may stay for days or weeks. If the urticaria is more pronounced and the reactions also extend to the deeper layers of the skin, swelling can occur. This swelling, being a consequence of an acute allergic reaction, and usually being in association with urticaria, is called **angioedema**.

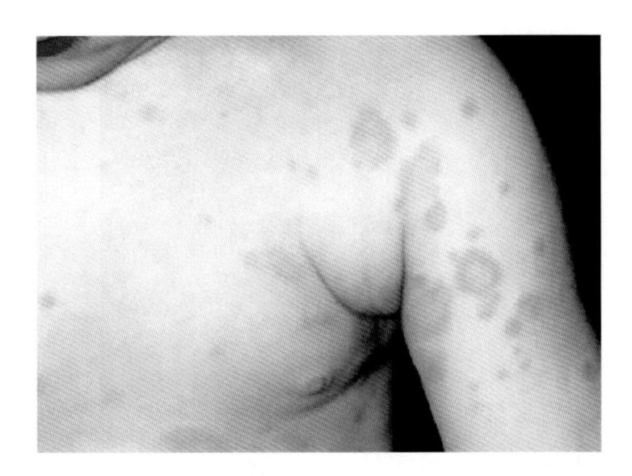

Fig. 1 Urticaria.

The incidence of urticaria and angioedema in a general population is 15-23%. In most cases, they present in combination, but they can also present separately. Data in children has shown that urticaria occurs in about 7% of non-selected preschool children and 17% of young children suffering from atopic dermatitis. Acute urticaria (Fig. 1) is more frequently seen in young people and children, and is linked to atopy or "allergic reactions", while chronic urticaria more frequently occurs in middle-aged, non-allergic women. If chronic urticaria is present in children, an underlying immunological or auto-immune disorder should be ruled out. A direct etiological cause can be suspected in more than 50% of acute urticaria, while this is only the case in about 20% for chronic urticaria.

Clinical presentation

Urticarial lesions or hives most commonly appear on the trunk, but may appear anywhere. The central area of superficial edema, or wheal, is surrounded by a variable amount of erythema, or

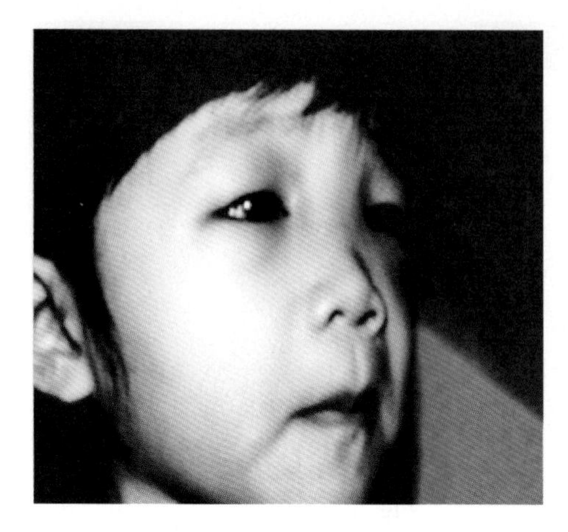

Fig. 2 Angioedema of eyes.

flare. This flare may be flat or have a raised border. Hives are almost always pruritic and may last from two to 48 hours. If pain is present, the diagnosis is more unlikely, and other diseases should be considered.

Angioedema (Fig. 2) is a deeper, less circumscribed swelling, which more frequently affects areas of loose connective tissue such as the face, eyelids, lips, tongue, and extremities. It is rarely pruritic, but may be painful, burning, or paresthetic. The time course of angioedema is similar to that of urticaria. Angioedema without urticaria can be the presentation of a rare hereditary disease, called C1 esterase inhibitor deficiency, which is mainly a disease of the complement system.

Classification

There is still some confusion on the classification of urticaria. Most authors divide it into three main types: acute, chronic, and physical (= induced by physical factors, such as pressure).

A. ACUTE URTICARIA

Acute urticaria has been defined as episodes lasting for less than six weeks (according to some authors, up to eight weeks or two months). It is the most frequent type of urticaria, especially in children and in atopics. Most patients have a single episode or only a few recurring episodes. There is often a specific cause, although one is not often readily identifiable. For one single episode, an extensive evaluation is hardly worthwhile.

B. CHRONIC URTICARIA

This form of urticaria has a peak incidence at ages 40 to 60 years, although children can also be affected. In adults, females are affected more than males, and no atopic association is demonstrable. A specific cause is identified in less than 20% of cases. In some cases, other organ systems may be involved, such as the gastrointestinal (nausea, vomiting, cramps, diarrhea), pulmonary (dyspnea), and musculoskeletal system (pain in joints and muscles). Malaise, fever, and headache may occur.

C. PHYSICAL URTICARIA

This includes a variety of syndromes induced by application of physical stimuli (pressure, water, temperature). The hives may be localized to the area of the stimulus, or they may be diffused. In most cases, urticaria develops within one half hour after the stimulus, although in rarer types such as delayed pressure urticaria, vibratory angioedema, and familial cold urticaria, the lesions may develop after several hours. In some cases, the involvement may be so diffused that anaphylaxis may result.

Differential diagnosis

There are several other skin disorders that should be considered in the evaluation of the child with urticaria and angioedema. Particularly, if the symptom *pruritus* is not present and is replaced by *pain*, the diagnosis of urticaria is very unlikely. *Urticaria* should be differentiated from:

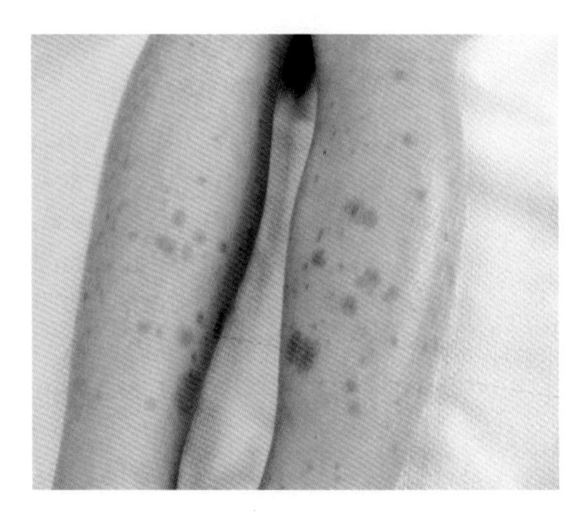

Fig. 3 Henoch – Schönlein purpura is a systemic vasculitis (inflammation in blood vessel wall). The lesions may affect the skin, the joints, the intestine and the kidneys. The skin lesions may resemble urticaria, but are usually non-itchy.

a. *Insect bites* (mosquitoes, gnats, ants). The lesions resemble hives, but are often associated with more local inflammation, can persist longer, and are often localized on the lower legs.
b. *Erythema multiforme.* May resemble urticaria in its earlier stages. However, the lesions last longer than 48 hours, often involve the palms and soles, and progress to blisters or target lesions.
c. *Henoch-Schönlein purpura* (HSP) (Fig.3) (and other types of *vasculitis*). Skin lesions in HSP may resemble urticaria. However, the symptoms/signs may include different types of skin bleeding (petechiae, purpura, peri-articular swelling), abdominal pain, and signs of renal involvement. Furthermore, in most subjects pruritus is absent.
d. *Scabies.* Can result in the appearance of pruritic erythematous papules or secondary urticaria.

Pruritus alone should be included in the differential diagnosis of urticaria. Generalized pruritus may be a manifestation of a systemic disease (Table 1).

Table 1 Diseases and Causes of Generalized Itch (pruritus)

- Xerosis (dry skin), types of eczema (including atopic dermatitis), allergic reactions
- Endocrine disorders: hyper- and hypothyroidism, diabetes mellitus, hyperparathyroidism
- Biliary obstruction, cholestasis
- Uremia
- Neoplasms: lymphoreticular, polycythemia vera, carcinoma, carcinoid syndrome
- Pregnancy
- Parasitic infestations
- Psychogenic

The differential diagnosis of angioedema includes *cellulitis (= a deep infection of the skin)*, as well as edema (swelling) from cardiac, renal, or hepatic disease. Other more uncommon possibilities also need to be considered.

Pathophysiology

The most important molecule that mediates urticaria and angioedema is **histamine**, stored in granules of **mast cells** (see Fig. 4). Injection of histamine in the skin results in the typical wheal and flare reaction of the urticarial lesion. In affected skin, an increased number of mast cells have been found. Mast cells, playing a pivotal role in the underlying mechanisms of urticaria, can be activated by IgE- or non-IgE-dependent mechanisms. They produce factors other than histamine, including tryptase, heparin, and many others. Through these mediators, mast cells can stimulate T-cell proliferation. T-cells also release different histamine-releasing factors as well as different cytokines, which can cause further mast cell and basophile degranulation through feedback loops. Recently, researchers focused on the role of ***blood basophils***, suggesting that

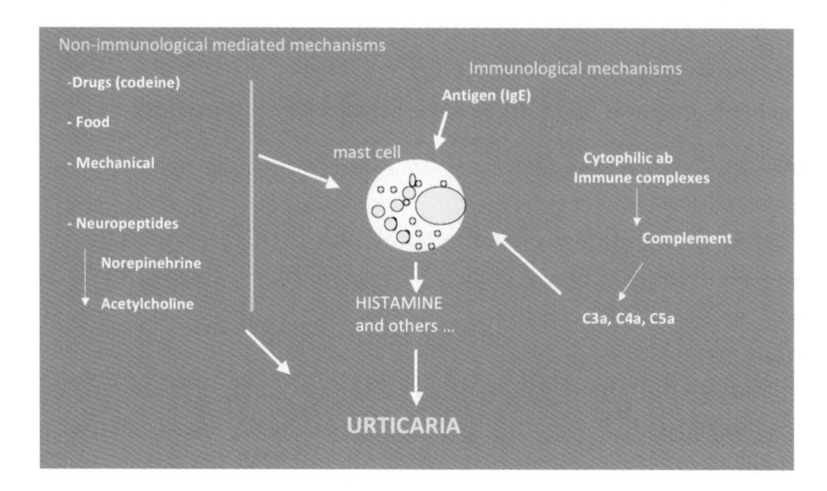

Fig. 4 Pathogenesis of urticaria. The central cell in urticaria and angioedema is the mast cell. Activation of mast cells leads to release of histamine (and other mediators), which is directly responsible for the symptoms of urticaria and angioedema. Mast cells can be activated by different mechanisms. Schematically, these mechanisms are divided into immunological and non-immunological triggers.

these cells may be recruited from the blood into urticarial wheals during disease activity.

Other mechanisms involved in urticaria are the production of ***IgG auto-antibodies, circulating immune complexes, and the activation of complement.***

Etiology of urticaria

In all types of urticaria, the underlying cause may be difficult to identify. In general, in only 50% of acute urticaria, can a cause be identified, while this is the case in about 20-30% of chronic urticaria. For *acute urticaria*, unless the reaction is severe or recurs frequently, an extensive evaluation is neither useful nor cost-effective. This is not the case in *chronic urticaria*, for which medications with their possible side effects justify a more aggressive attempt to find an avoidable or treatable etiology.

Table 2 Possible Causes of Urticaria and Angioedema

Drugs	Infections
Foods and food additives	Collagen-vascular disease
Insect bites and stings	Malignancy (myeloid leukemia)
Contactants	Vasculitis
Immunotherapy	C1 esterase inhibitor deficiency
Inhalants	Physical urticaria
Systemic diseases	
Endocrine disease	

Furthermore, chronic urticaria can be an early manifestation of a severe systemic disease in children, needing early and aggressive treatment. In Table 2, a list is given of categories of etiologic factors to consider in the evaluation of children with chronic and acute urticaria.

DRUGS

Drugs are the most common identifiable cause of urticaria. Almost any drug is capable of inducing urticaria by IgE- or non-IgE-mediated mechanisms. A well-known example is *penicillin*, being able to induce urticaria via IgE-mediated allergic mechanisms or through a serum sickness syndrome. Other drugs are capable of activating mast cells directly. These include morphine, codeine, curare, polymyxin B, vancomycin, thiamine, doxorubicin, and radiocontrast dye.

Approximately 20-40% of adult patients with urticaria or angioedema will experience exacerbations with *aspirin* or other non-steroidal anti-inflammatory agents (NSAIDS). The prevalence in children is lower, although the exact percentage is unknown.

FOOD and FOOD ADDITIVES

Food and food additives are other commonly encountered causes of urticaria, especially acute urticaria in *children* and in *atopic individuals*. Only occasionally, food and food additives have been shown to be important in chronic urticaria. Reactions are usually IgE-mediated, but non-IgE-mediated mechanisms also do

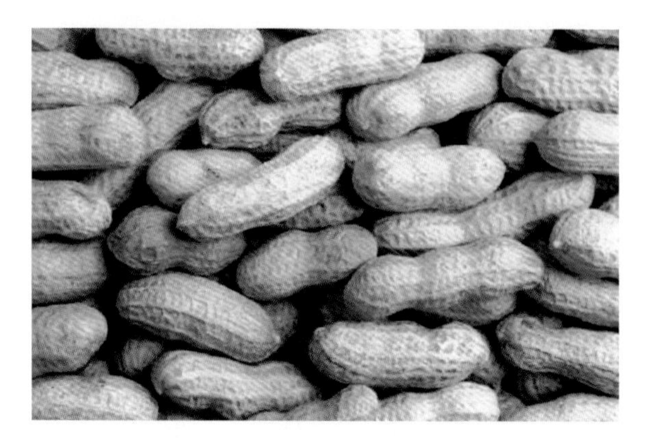

Fig. 5 A common manifestation of peanut allergy is acute urticaria.

occur. Among the IgE-mediated reactions are the reactions to peanuts (Fig. 5) (which can be life-threatening), nuts, seafood, wheat, soybeans and fruits (cfr. cross-reactivity with latex), such as banana, kiwi, and lychee.

In a recent study it was suggested that sensitization to peanut protein may occur in children through the application of peanut oil to inflamed skin. These findings could lead to new strategies to prevent sensitization in infants at risk. Non-IgE-mediated urticaria to food by direct mast cell activation, include reactions to tomatoes, strawberries, shellfish, and mussels.

Several anecdotal reports and uncontrolled studies implicated various preservatives (benzoates, sulfites), food dyes (tartrazine, coal-tar derivates), yeasts (Candida, baker's), natural substances (salicylates), and flavorings (MSG, saccharin) as causes of acute and chronic reactions. Reactions were more frequently described in adults than in children. However, in some children suffering from severe eczema, flares of eczema and urticaria were observed after double-blind provocation with food additives. Therefore, there is no doubt that these reactions can occur, but much less frequently than has been suggested, as shown in a very elegant study in adults with chronic urticaria and atopic dermatitis, using double-blind, placebo-controlled challenge tests. The results of the study

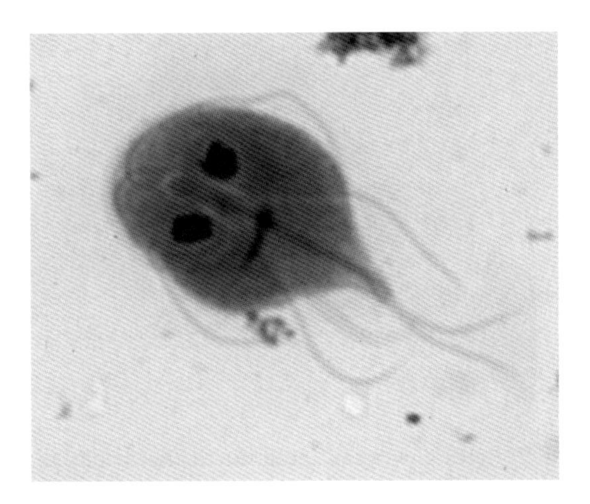

Fig. 6 *Giardia lamblia* is an intestinal parasite that can cause diarrhea. However, some children carry this parasite without any symptoms of diarrhea or tummy pain. In these children the parasite can induce chronic urticaria.

clearly demonstrate that common food additives **are seldom if ever** of significance as precipitating factors in chronic urticaria or atopic dermatitis. In another study, using placebo-controlled oral challenges, no more than 10% of patients with chronic urticaria had confirmed reactions to food additives.

INFECTIOUS CAUSES

Infectious causes are common in acute urticaria, not in chronic urticaria. Some reports have related chronic urticaria to occult chronic bacterial infections, such as dental abscesses or vaginal infections, but these are uncommon. Other infections associated with urticaria include ECHO, coxsachie virus, a parvo B19 virus, EBV, *Mycoplasma pneumonia* and cytomegalovirus. Although an association between chronic urticaria and infestation with helminthes (*Ascaria*, *Trichinella*, *Schistosoma*) and protozoa (ameba, *Giardia*, *Trichomonas*) has been described, it is rare even in endemic areas. In young children attending day-care centers, an association between acute urticaria and *Giardia lamblia* (Fig. 6) infection of the intestine has been described.

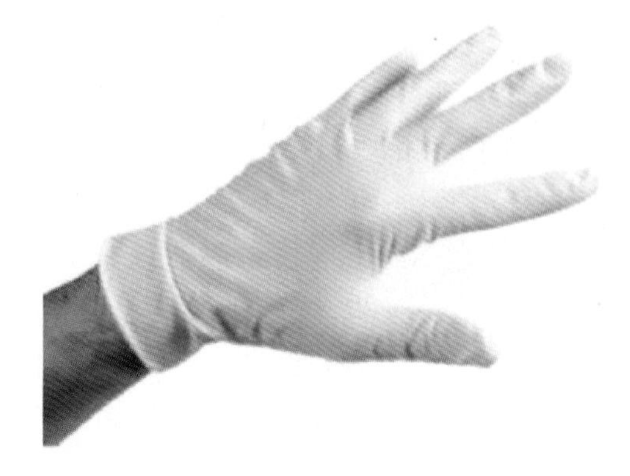

Fig. 7 Latex gloves can induce urticaria. Especially, children with spina bifida are very prone to developing latex allergy, due to early and repeated contacts with latex.

INSECT BITES AND STINGS

Insect bites or insect stings may appear as papular urticaria in children. These lesions can represent part of a systemic reaction to Hymenoptera or fire ants and may warrant evaluation and possible immunotherapy.

CONTACT URTICARIA

This is seen in highly sensitive individuals and has been described with latex, animals (cfr. urticaria after animal bites, such as bites from hamsters), food (cross-reactivity between birch pollen and fruit), plants, sea nettles, and caterpillars. Industrial chemicals, medications, and cosmetics can also cause contact urticaria.

Urticaria after exposure to **latex** (Fig. 7) has been described extensively, especially in children with spina bifida. Exposure can occur via many routes – cutaneous, percutaneous, mucosal, and parenteral. Furthermore, the antigens can be transferred either directly or via aerosol transmission. Cutaneous and respiratory exposure has been shown to invoke severe systemic reactions, but direct mucosal and parenteral exposure poses the greatest risk of anaphylaxis.

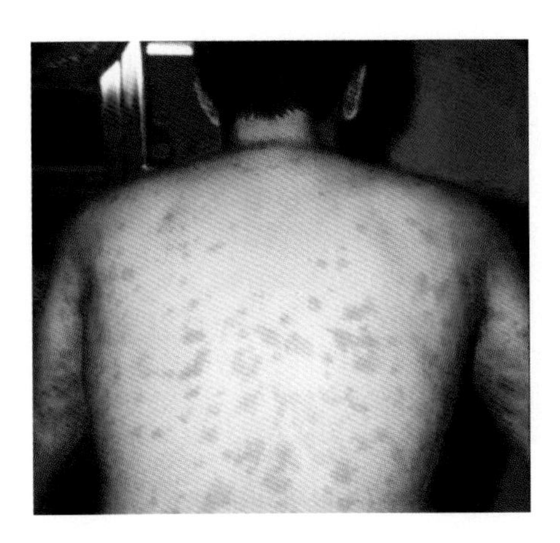

Fig. 8 Physical urticaria after exercise in an adolescent.

Inhalant allergens may, in rare instances, result in urticaria, and usually with the association of respiratory symptoms. Nevertheless, individuals extremely allergic to inhalants, such as grass pollen, may develop urticaria on contact with these specific allergens.

SYSTEMIC DISEASES

A number of systemic diseases may present as chronic urticaria in children. The major disease categories of systemic diseases include: infections, connective tissue disease (such as systemic lupus erythematosus (SLE) and others), endocrine dysfunction (hyper- and hypothyroidism, diabetes, and others), and malignancy (myeloid leukemia, non-Hodgkin's lymphoma, and others).

Physical urticaria

Physical urticaria (Fig. 8) is triggered by a specific "physical" stimulus. This type of urticaria is rather common, affecting 17% of all urticaria patients, especially children and young adults. Lesions usually appear within 30 minutes of exposure to the stimulus and

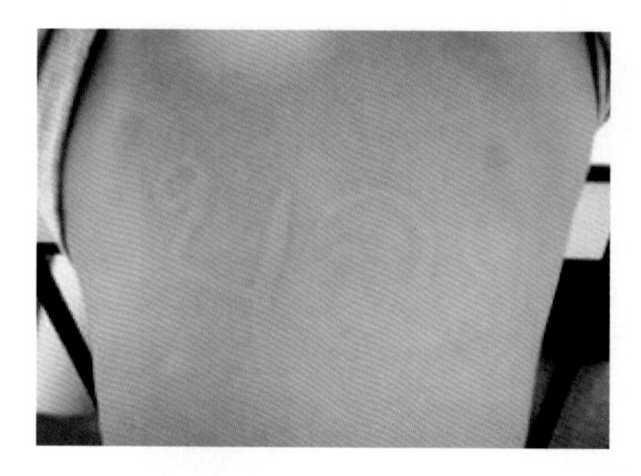

Fig. 9 Dermographism.

are often limited to the areas of stimuli. **Mast cell degranulation** seems to be the central event, and mast cell mediators, especially histamine, were found in venous blood draining and in tissue taken from affected sites. The exact mechanism by which a physical stimulus results in mast cell activation is not well understood, but might be linked to a congenital ability of mast cells to degranulate.

TYPES OF PHYSICAL URTICARIA

a. Dermographism (Fig. 9)

This is the most common type of physical urticaria, occurring in up to 5% of the general population, especially in young children and infants (after bathing, after sweating). Girls seem to be more frequently affected than boys.

b. Pressure-induced urticaria

Apart from dermographism, other distinct forms of pressure-induced lesions have been described. They occur often in children with chronic urticaria in areas of pressure (cfr. belt lines) in the absence of demonstrable dermographism. A variant is **"delayed pressure urticaria (DPU)"**, originally described as a rare familial disorder, but now also recognized in some patients with chronic urticaria. Lesions are erythematous, swollen, and painful and develop four to six hours following a pressure stimulus. DPU can be mistaken as angioedema. A variant of DPU is **hereditary**

(autosomal dominant) vibratory angioedema (i.e. urticaria following motorcycling, etc). DPU is usually unresponsive to antihistamines. Some patients respond to NSAIDs and a considerable number of adult patients will require daily corticosteroids, often in moderate doses.

c. Cholinergic urticaria

This occurs in up to 7% of all forms of urticaria, especially in teenagers and young adults. The lesions are induced by exercise, "core heating", sweating, and emotional stress. The characteristic lesions are small, punctuate, highly pruritic, and surrounded by extensive erythema. The nervous system effector mechanisms involved in the compensatory responses in thermoregulation may lead to mast cell activation. Treatment involves the avoidance of exogenous heat provocation, cooling, and the usage of antihistamines, particularly hydroxizin or cetirizine.

d. Exercise-induced urticaria/ anaphylaxis

This type of urticaria differs from cholinergic urticaria in that raising the core temperature in the absence of exercise will *not* provoke an attack. Additionally, the lesions are usually larger.

e. Temperature-related urticaria

- Heat-induced urticaria usually falls under the category of cholinergic urticaria, although a rare subset has been described in which the local application of heat will cause an isolated urticarial eruption.
- Cold urticaria is more common and may be life-threatening. Deaths have been described in patients who dived into cold water. Cold-induced urticaria may be either familial (autosomal dominant) or acquired (essential). Acquired cold urticaria may develop following insect stings, viral infections, drug reactions, or even after childbirth.

f. Other types of physical urticaria

- *Adrenergic urticaria*, developing at times of stress, has been described. The lesions are widespread, pruritic, papular, and surrounded by a striking white halo.

- *Solar urticaria* is rare in children and occurs usually within 30 minutes of sun exposure. This type of urticaria can be associated with drug ingestion (tetracycline), insect stings, infection, and underlying systemic diseases such as systemic lupus erythematosus.
- *Aquagenic urticaria*, a very rare disorder, results from contact with water. Clinically, the lesions are indistinguishable from cholinergic urticaria. Some patients can have both forms. In one study it was suggested that a water-soluble epidermal antigen permeates the skin in the presence of water and activates cutaneous mast cells. Therapy includes inert skin oils and antihistamines.

Treatment of urticaria

Except for the patients for whom an avoidable cause can be identified (such as food), treatment of urticaria is symptomatic. The medication of first choice to treat all types of urticaria is an antihistamine. Some investigators advocate avoiding certain medications (such as aspirin and other NSAIDs) in all patients suffering from **chronic** urticaria, but this approach has never been proven for children.

Treatment depends on the severity of symptoms. Scattered or mild hives are self-limited and usually require no treatment, or at most, a mild ***antihistamine*** as needed. In a number of comparative trials between the various non-sedating agents (*loratadine, desloratidine, cetirizine, and levocetirizine)*, no significant difference in efficacy has been noted. All the agents have good safety profiles in children. However, in young children the situation is less evident. Only a limited number of antihistamines have been studied on efficacy and safety in young children. The most extensive safety studies in young children were done with cetirizine and levocetirizine. Ketotifen has also been studied in infants, but less extensively.

In cases of severe urticaria or angioedema, treatment should be similar to that of an anaphylactic reaction (i.e. shock) (Chapter 10).

The first choice of medication for urticaria is antihistamines.

Topical medications (creams) containing corticosteroids, topical antihistamines, and local anesthetics have no role in the management.

In addition to antihistamines, the mainstay of therapy in severe cases is ***subcutaneous epinephrine***, while corticosteroid therapy is rarely necessary. Some patients suffering from recurrent urticaria with known cause (i.e. food, or insect stings) should be encouraged to carry and be trained to use injectable epinephrine (such as Epipen).

Conclusion

Urticaria in children remains a difficult and frustrating problem, as in most children no cause can be identified, especially in those children suffering from chronic urticaria.

For **acute urticaria**, diagnostic investigations are rarely necessary, except in those few patients with life-threatening disease (cfr. anaphylactic reactions). A carefully taken history still remains the most important tool to identify a possible trigger (i.e. food and medication).

Most children suffering from **chronic urticaria** deserve a diagnostic work-up. In these children, it is important to exclude underlying systemic diseases for which early treatment is necessary.

8 Food Allergy

Food allergy (FA) is a difficult and confusing issue, mainly because FA is surrounded with many stories, non-scientific data and superstition, leading to misdiagnosis. Furthermore, the concepts of FA are understood wrongly, and therefore, approached wrongly by many people. Often parents come to the clinic requesting to test their child for food allergy, because the child has symptoms such as bad school results, sleep problems or stomach pain, and they suspect the cause to be food. Most of these children are not food allergic, and other causes (often psychological causes) are involved. Sometimes parents persist in their search for FA, ending up with all kinds of non-scientific diagnostic tests and extensive diets, leading to malnutrition and more psychological distress in the child.

Obtaining an accurate picture of the burden of FA is hampered by the lack of uniform, population-based methodologies that incorporate the gold-standard diagnostic method (see below: a double-blind, placebo-controlled oral food challenge). For example, self-reported FA ranged from 3% to 35%, which likely reflects study limitations of self-report, varied definitions of FA, and true population variation. Prevalence studies based on the incorporation of appropriate food challenges are limited. However, based on these criteria, the true prevalence of FA is estimated to be between 1% and 11%, being higher in children than in adults. While it seems that FA is increasing worldwide, it also should be considered that methodological issues in various studies differ, and therefore, we should be cautious with the interpretation of results.

FA should be approached scientifically. Only this approach will help children and parents appropriately, and will avoid useless interventions (extensive diets) and useless spending of money, as some of the diagnostic tests are very expensive.

Parts of FA have been covered in the previous chapters and will not be repeated here (see listing).

LISTING OF CHAPTERS & PAGES IN WHICH PARTS OF FOOD ALLERGY WERE COVERED

Chapter 1: Listing of food allergens (pages 2)
Chapter 2: Epidemiology of FA (pages 32)
Chapter 3: Coverage of the important food allergens (pages 44)
Chapter 6: The role of food in eczema (pages 110)
Chapter 7: The role of food as causes of urticaria and angioedema (pages 140)

Definition of food allergy

Any abnormal reaction that results from the ingestion of food is considered an ***adverse food reaction***. Critical to any discussion on adverse food reactions is a basic understanding of the classification of the different reactions to food. The utilization of these terms will allow better communication regarding various reactions to food components.

A number of types of adverse reactions are distinguished (Table 1). The terminology is not always clear, as different researchers use different definitions. Usually adverse reactions to food are divided into three groups: **food intolerance, food allergy** (including IgE-mediated reactions) and **food aversions or phobias**. Most researchers consider the term "food allergy" as an abnormal reaction from the human body in which the immune system is involved. The term "food allergy" is used in this chapter for all abnormal immunological reactions, not only for the IgE-mediated reactions. This definition is therefore different from all other allergic reactions, pointing to the involvement of IgE. Any abnormal reaction to food in which the immune system is not involved is **not** considered as food allergic reactions.

Table 1 Three Types of Adverse Reactions to Food

1. Food intolerance
2. Food allergy
3. Food aversion

1. FOOD INTOLERANCE

Food intolerance is **the most common type of adverse reaction to foods**. It is a general term describing an abnormal physiological response to an ingested food. A number of underlying causes have been identified, which may be due to either the food or the host. Usually, the symptoms are diarrhea, stomach pain, and vomiting. The most common types are:

a. Intolerance caused by toxic contaminants of food

Examples: High histamine in scombroid fish poisoning, toxins from bacteria, such as Salmonella, Shigella, and Campylobacter.

b. Intolerance caused by pharmacologic properties of the food

Examples: Alcohol, caffeine in coffee, tyramine in aged cheeses, or food poisoning by

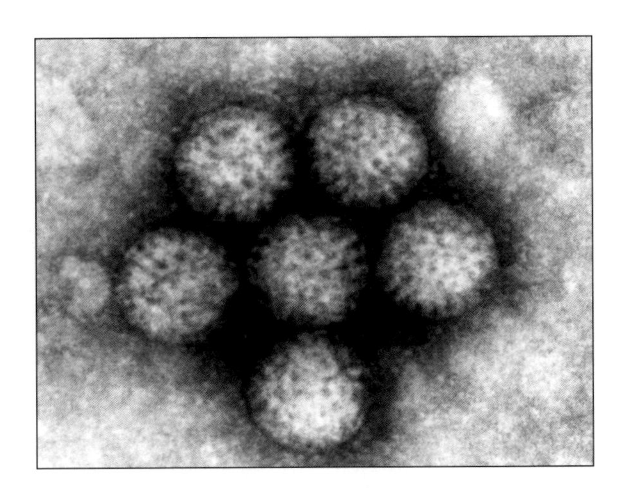

Fig. 1 Rotavirus is the most common cause of acute diarrhea in children, worldwide. Recently a vaccine has been launched against the virus, showing good effectiveness.

foods containing heavy metals or pesticides.

c. Intolerance caused by infected food

Examples: Food containing bacteria, parasites, or viruses (Fig. 1) (such as rotavirus infection, by drinking contaminated water)

d. Intolerance caused by characteristics of the host

Example: Metabolic disorders, such as lactase deficiency, causing intolerance to milk.

2. FOOD ALLERGY

Food allergy is more common in young children. This type of reaction may occur after only a small amount of the food is ingested, and is unrelated to any physiologic effect of the food. Usually, food allergy is caused by an underlying IgE-mediated hypersensitivity reaction, but other types of immunological reactions have been identified. Food allergic reactions include:

1. IgE-mediated reactions
2. Non-IgE-mediated reactions

Food allergy is a difficult subject, and parents usually don't have the expertise to make a diagnosis themselves (although they have the best intentions for their child).

This results often in situations in which children are given extensive and unnecessary diets, which may induce various types of malnutrition. If a parent suspects that her/his child suffers from a food allergy, it is advised to seek specialized medical assistance.

Various types have been identified, including cellular-mediated mechanisms (involving T-lymphocytes; these reactions have a delayed onset), mixed types (involving IgE and cells, such as in eczema), and other mechanisms constituting a large variety of reactions. Of some, the underlying mechanisms are unknown. In some, immune complexes or complement are involved.

3. FOOD AVERSION

Food aversions or food phobias are psychological reactions that may mimic food allergy. Moreover, some children who are food allergic will refuse the foods that cause allergic reactions. Sometimes distinguishing food allergy from food aversion is very difficult, and parents should not persist to give food that has caused symptoms in their children. Typically, real food aversion cannot be reproduced when the child ingests the food in a blinded fashion.

- Apart from the above different types of adverse food reactions, a number of underlying diseases can mimic food allergy. There is a long list of diseases, of which the most common are: diseases of the gastrointestinal tract (pyloric stenosis, hiatal hernia, diseases of the liver, gallbladder, pancreas) and enzyme deficiencies or metabolic diseases.

Food allergic reactions are abnormal reactions to food in which the immune system is involved. Different underlying mechanisms of food allergy can be distinguished. The most important are:

1. <u>IgE-mediated reactions</u>
   = best studied model, causing the most severe reactions to food.

2. <u>Immune complexes mediated reactions</u>
   = involving complexes of food antigens and IgG antibodies, that can induce adverse reactions by activating inflammatory cells and the complement system. Also called type III reactions

3. <u>Cell-mediated reactions</u>
   = mediated by lymphocytes and also referred to as delayed reactions of type IV reactions

Fig 2. Mechanisms of food allergy.

Mechanisms of food allergy

A. IgE-MEDIATED FOOD ALLERGY

This type of reaction has been extensively described in previous chapters (see Chapter 1 on "Allergy and Allergic Reactions"). In short, these reactions occur in genetically predisposed patients and are the result of an excessive production of food-specific IgE antibodies. These antibodies bind (through receptors) on different cells, such as mast cells, basophiles, and other cells. After the food allergens reach the food-specific IgE antibodies on mast cells and basophiles, various mediators such as histamine, prostaglandins, and leukotrienes are released. These mediators then induce different symptoms of immediate hypersensitivity. The activated mast cells may also release various cytokines that play a part in inflammatory reactions (also called late-phase reactions).

B. NON-IgE-MEDIATED FOOD ALLERGY

A large variety of non-IgE-mediated types of FA have been described (Fig. 2). However, these types are much less documented than the IgE-mediated type, and therefore, the scientific evidence supporting these mechanisms is limited. The most important types of non-IgE-mediated food allergic reactions are:

- Type III reactions involving immune complexes (= soluble antigen-antibody complexes that affect functioning of different organs) have been described. However, there is little support from systematic studies that these complexes are able to mediate FA.
- Type IV reactions (i.e. cell-mediated reactions, also called delayed type of hypersensitivity) has been suggested in several disorders where the clinical symptoms do not appear until several hours after intake of the suspected food. This type of immune response may contribute to some food allergic reactions (such as enterocolitis) but significant supporting evidence of a specific cell-mediated hypersensitivity disorder is lacking.
- Mixed types involving IgE and cellular hypersensitivity reactions have been suggested and some researchers consider these mixed types of reactions to be involved in atopic dermatitis. Recently, a role of Th17 (a newly discovered type of T-helper lymphocytes, which can drive inflammatory reactions) has been attributed to these types of reactions.

Symptoms of FA, and symptoms that are not caused by FA

The most common clinical presentation of an IgE-mediated FA is **the sudden appearance of urticaria (hives), within minutes after intake of a food, such as peanuts, seafood, or fish**. (Table 2) In more severe cases, there is also presence of angioedema, presenting itself as swelling of the lips or eyes. When the FA is really very severe (Fig. 3), symptoms of difficult respiration (asthma, difficult breathing) and even anaphylactic shock (drop in blood pressure and coma) can appear, being potentially fatal and needing urgent treatment.

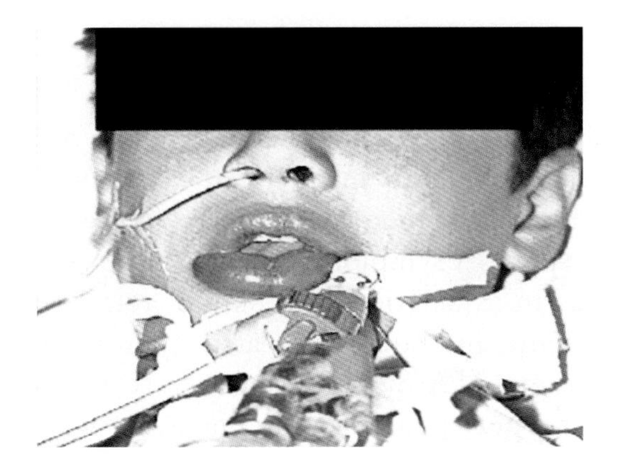

Fig. 3 Severe angioedema, needing artificial ventilation, caused by food allergy in a 10-year-old child (Courtesy of Prof. Gideon Lack, London).

Table 2 Sequence of a Typical "full blown" IgE-mediated Food Allergic Reaction

Itch (neck, trunk)
↓
Urticaria (spreading over the whole body)
↓
Swelling of lips – eyes
↓
Swelling of tongue – itchy throat
↓
Difficult breathing – wheezing + rhinitis (sneezing) + conjunctivitis
↓
Fainting – coma – anaphylactic shock

A. SYMPTOMS OF IgE-MEDIATED FOOD ALLERGY

1. Skin and respiratory food allergic reactions

The skin is the most frequently target organ in IgE-mediated FA. The ingestion of food allergens can induce either immediate cutaneous symptoms or aggravate chronic symptoms (such as eczema). Acute urticaria and angioedema are the most common manifestations of FA, generally appearing within minutes of ingestion of the food allergen.

Respiratory symptoms usually appear in association with skin symptoms, and rarely as isolated symptoms of FA. Symptoms may include peri-ocular erythema (rash surrounding the eyes), itchy eyes, tearing, nasal congestion (blocked nose), sneezing, runny nose, cough, voice changes, and wheezing and difficult breathing.

A very well-described entity in this group is the oral allergy syndrome (OAS).

OAS (Fig. 4) is considered a form of **contact urticaria** induced by exposure of the oral and pharyngeal mucosa to food allergens, being a consequence of **a cross-reactivity between certain foods and inhaled allergens.** The syndrome is classified by some researchers under the group of gastrointestinal symptoms of FA. Affected patients may present with rapid onset of symptoms with increasing severity, from mild itching of the lips, mouth and throat, to lip and tongue swelling, to severe angioedema of the throat (pharyngeal mucosa) up to life-threatening emergencies, such as anaphylaxis. OAS is an important alarm manifestation in subjects at risk for severe allergic reactions. Generally, OAS is related to plant-derived foods only, but also severe reactions to animal-derived foods may be preceded and accompanied by local oral symptoms. The triggering food may be dependent on geographically different nutritional habits and may thus vary from place to place. Patients with allergic rhinitis to certain airborne pollen (especially birch, mugwort and ragweed) are frequently afflicted with OAS (Europe, USA, seldom in Asia). Patients with birch pollen sensitization often have symptoms following the ingestion of stone fruits and pip fruits, but also after vegetables such as carrots or celery, nuts, legumes. Patients with ragweed pollen sensitization may experience allergic symptoms following contact with certain melons (watermelon, cantaloupe, honeydew, etc) and bananas.

Other examples are:

- Allergy to seafood in patients with house dust mite allergy
- Allergy to vegetables and fruits in patients with latex allergy (such as in children with spina bifida)

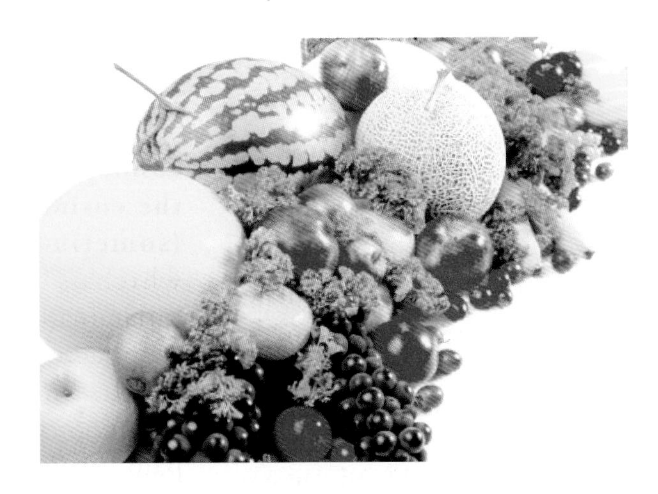

Fig. 4 Oral allergy syndrome (OAS) occurs as a consequence of cross-reactivity between pollen and vegetables or fruits. These patients will suffer from allergic rhinitis during the pollen season, and also of urticaria – angioedema after eating certain vegetables or fruits.

2. Gastrointestinal symptoms of FA

IgE-mediated gastrointestinal symptoms of FA include immediate gastrointestinal hypersensitivity and allergic eosinophilic gastroenteritis.

- *Immediate gastrointestinal hypersensitivity*

This type of hypersensitivity may accompany allergic symptoms in other organs. The symptoms vary but may include nausea, abdominal pain, abdominal cramping, vomiting, and/or diarrhea. Symptoms may resemble those of a gastrointestinal infection and need to be distinguished from it. Complete elimination of the suspected food allergen for up to two weeks will lead to a resolution of symptoms. Diagnosis is usually made by a food challenge, although positive skin prick tests suggest FA. Foods that have been associated with immediate gastrointestinal hypersensitivity are milk, egg, peanut, soy, cereal, and fish.

- ***Allergic eosinophilic gastroenteritis***

This type of FA is a mixed IgE-mediated and non-IgE-mediated type of FA. It is a disorder characterized by infiltration of the gastric and/or intestinal wall with eosinophils and raised numbers of eosinophils in the blood. Patients presenting with this syndrome frequently have post-prandial nausea and vomiting, abdominal pain, diarrhea, failure to thrive, or weight loss. Diagnosis is difficult, and is usually based upon an appropriate history and a gastrointestinal biopsy demonstrating a characteristic eosinophilic infiltration. However, multiple biopsies may be needed because the eosinophilic infiltrates may be quite patchy. Patients with this disease usually have other atopic symptoms (eczema), including multiple food allergic reactions, elevated IgE levels, positive skin prick tests and blood eosinophilia. In other patients, anemia and low levels of proteins in the blood (hypoalbuminemia) can be found. An elimination diet of up to 12 weeks may be necessary before the complete resolution of symptoms occurs.

A separate entity, related to eosinophilic gastroenteritis, is **the eosinophilic oesphagitis (sometimes with gastritis)**, which is a chronic allergic inflammatory condition of the esophagus, which most often results in dysphagia, bolus impaction, heartburn, or chest pain. Of particular importance is the differentiation from other inflammatory diseases of the esophagus, especially gastro-esophageal reflux disease. Biopsies from the proximal to the distal esophagus demonstrating >15-20 eosinophils per field favor the diagnosis. Besides avoidance of the responsible food allergens, common treatment regimens in children and adults involve also the ingestion of topical corticosteroids.

B. SYMPTOMS OF NON-IgE-MEDIATED FOOD ALLERGY

A large variety of non-IgE-mediated food allergic disorders has been described. Usually, these disorders are much less documented than the IgE-mediated type of FA. Among the many disorders, the most important are:

1. Dietary protein enterocolitis (also called protein intolerance)

This is a rare disease of young infants, usually starting between the ages of one week and three months. The typical symptoms are isolated to the gastrointestinal tract and consist of recurrent vomiting and/or diarrhea. The symptoms can be severe, causing dehydratation. The disease is usually associated with a non-IgE-mediated allergy to cow's milk or soy milk, while in older infants egg has been reported to be responsible for the disease. Elimination of the offending food allergen generally will result in improvement or resolution of symptoms within 72 hours. Skin prick tests or determination of specific IgE in the blood are negative. Diagnosis is based on an oral food challenge, which can result in severe symptoms. The disease usually settles by the age of 18-24 months.

2. Dietary protein proctitis – colitis

This disease usually presents during the first months of life and is often secondary to cow's milk or soy protein hypersensitivity, affecting the large intestinal and terminal intestinal segment. Infants with this disorder often do not appear ill, have normally formed stools, and generally are discovered because of the presence of blood in their stools. It is accepted, without well-controlled studies, that the disease resolves by age six months to two years of allergen avoidance.

The disease can also appear in infants who are fully breast-fed, through foreign proteins (usually cow's milk proteins) that are present in breast milk (dependent on the mother's diet).

3. Celiac disease

Celiac disease is an extensive enteropathy leading to malabsorption and failure to thrive. Total villous atrophy (destruction of small intestine) and an extensive cellular infiltrate are associated with sensitivity to the alcohol-soluble portion of **gluten** found in wheat, oat, rye, and barley. This is also called **gluten intolerance**. Gluten is found mainly in foods but may also be found in products we use every day, such as stamp and envelope adhesive, medicines, and vitamins. Because the body's own immune system causes the damage,

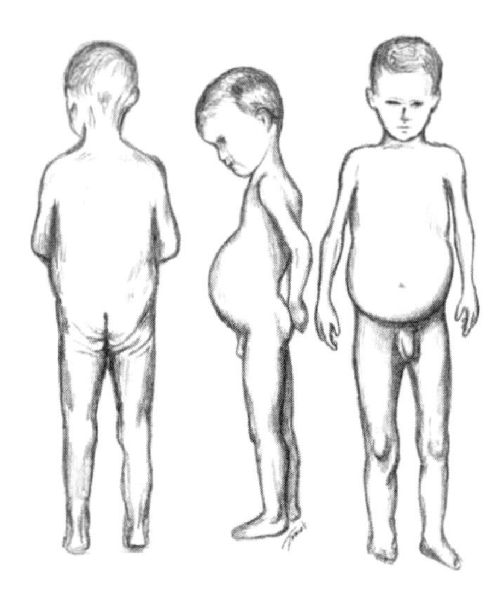

Fig. 5 Celiac disease: is a malabsorption caused by gluten intolerance. Children often have symptoms of chronic diarrhea, abdominal distention, and failure to thrive.

celiac disease is considered an autoimmune disorder. However, it is also classified as a disease of malabsorption because nutrients are not absorbed. Celiac disease (Fig. 5) is also known as celiac sprue, non-tropical sprue, and gluten-sensitive enteropathy. It is a genetic disease, meaning it runs in families. Sometimes the disease is triggered — or becomes active for the first time — after surgery, pregnancy, childbirth, viral infection, or severe emotional stress. Patients often have presenting symptoms of diarrhea or "steatorrhea" (fatty stools), abdominal distention and flatulence, weight loss, and occasionally nausea and vomiting. However, a person with celiac disease may have no symptoms. People without symptoms are still at risk for the complications of celiac disease, including malnutrition. The longer a patient goes undiagnosed and untreated, the greater the chance of developing malnutrition and other complications. Anemia, delayed growth, and weight loss are signs of malnutrition: the body is just not getting enough nutrients.

Manifestations of the skin, the respiratory tract, and the gastrointestinal tract are the most common symptoms of food allergy. Symptoms resulting from other organs (especially psychological or neurological symptoms) are usually not due to food allergy!

C. SYMPTOMS THAT ARE (USUALLY) NOT CAUSED BY FOOD ALLERGY

FA usually manifests itself through reactions from the skin (urticaria, eczema), the respiratory tract (rhinitis, asthma), or the gastrointestinal tract (vomiting, diarrhea). Diseases from other organs (kidney, brain, heart, etc) are usually not due to food allergy, especially neurological or psychological disorders. However, often parents believe that FA is involved in their child's problems. Neurological, psychological, or psychiatric diseases are usually not caused by FA. These include: sleep or learning problems, hyperactivity, autism, and migraine.

Foods that cause food allergy and their geographic aspects

In theory, worldwide, all foods can cause food allergy, as foods contain proteins that are considered foreign by the human immune system and might induce IgE production in all human beings with an underlying, genetically-determined allergic constitution.

However, most food allergic reactions are caused by a limited number of foods, are age specific, and have their own geographical distribution. In general, in young children FA is mainly caused by cow's milk, hen's egg, soy, and wheat. In older children, FA is

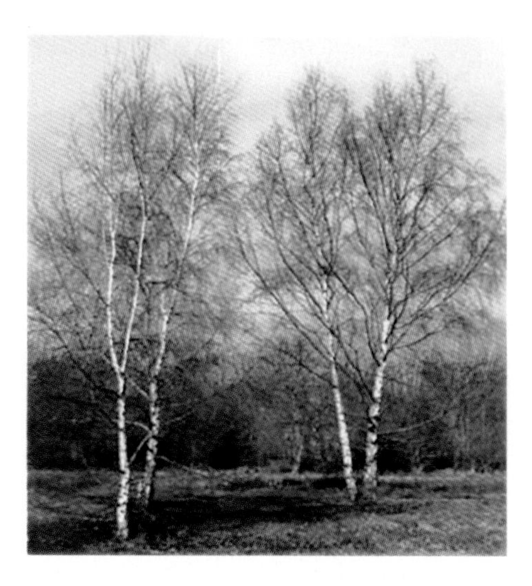

Fig. 6 Birch pollen allergy is a main cause of food allergy (through cross-reactivity) in Central and Northern Europe, leading to the oral allergy syndrome (OAS). The immunological basis of this phenomenon is IgE cross-reactivity due to highly homologous amino acid sequences resulting in homologous structures of pollen and food allergens of plant origin.

usually caused by seafood, peanut, fish, and fruits or vegetables (cfr. OSA). Extensive coverage of the different foods that can cause FA is given in Chapter 3.

The list of the most prevalent triggering foods leading to allergic reactions in different geographic areas show important differences that may be most likely explained by **different nutritional habits** or by **differences in exposure to inhalant allergens** (see below: birch pollen (Fig. 6) and OAS). Whereas in the USA, UK, and Scandinavian countries, peanuts and nuts are the most prevalent elicitors of anaphylaxis to foods, but this is not the case in other regions. In France, for instance, egg and seafood, in Switzerland, celery (a pollen-related food), or in Australia, seafood, are the top culprit foods for potentially life threatening allergic reactions to foods.

In Central and Northern Europe, FA of plant origin is in most instances mediated by sensitization to **birch pollen**, and up to 80% of birch pollen allergic patients suffer from an associated food allergy (cfr. OAS).

Birch pollen sensitized patients are mainly affected by allergic reactions to foods of the *Rosaceae*

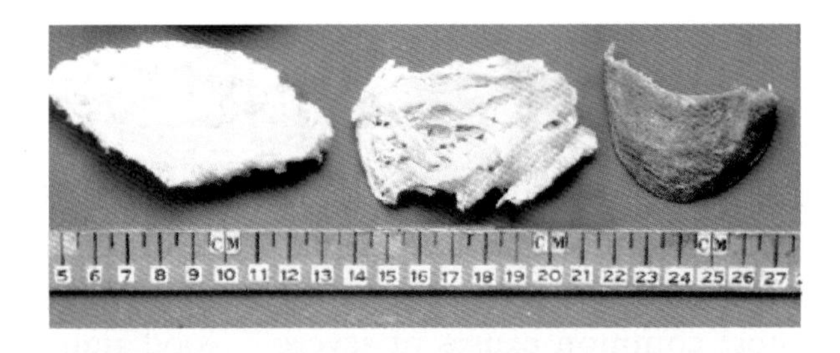

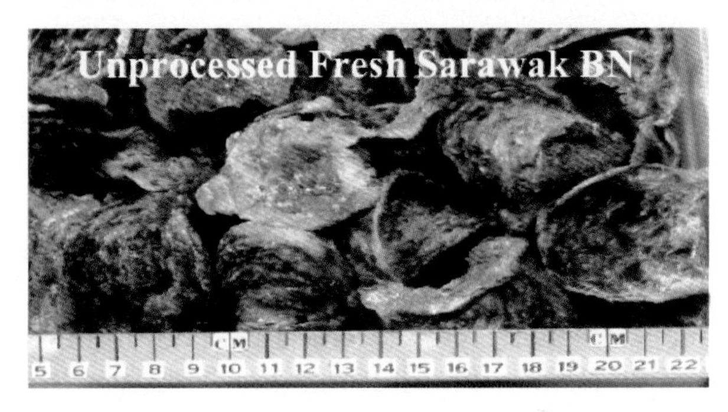

Fig. 7 Bird's nest allergy is one of the most common causes of severe food allergy in Singapore, which can lead to anaphylaxis. Bird's nest is a popular Chinese delicacy believed to have health benefits.

family such as apple, pear, cherry, and nectarine, but also to kiwi and various vegetables or nuts. The immunological basis of this phenomenon is IgE cross-reactivity due to highly homologous amino acid sequences resulting in homologous structures of pollen and food allergens of plant origin.

FOOD ALLERGY IN ASIA

Only a few population-based studies on FA in Asia have been published. Prevalences of FA in Asian children were found to be 4% in Singapore and rural China, to as high as 12% in Seoul, Korea, and Japan. The exact reason for this wide range in prevalence is not known, but could mirror that these differences are related to survey methodologies rather than a true difference.

Furthermore, it has been observed that certain specific foods consumed mainly in the Asian region have resulted in allergies that are unique to their respective populations. An example of this is that allergy to **bird's nest** (Fig. 7) from swiftlets has been described in the Chinese population in Singapore, Malaysia, and Hong Kong. It is one of the most common causes of severe FA, leading to anaphylaxis in Singapore children. Bird's nest is a popular Chinese delicacy believed to have health benefits.

Similarly, **royal jelly**, another food that is very popular amongst the Chinese, has also been reported to trigger asthma and anaphylaxis in Hong Kong and in ethnic Chinese in Australia. **Buckwheat** causing anaphylaxis has been observed in Japan, Korea, and China. Buckwheat is consumed in large quantities by these populations in the form of noodles or soba. Similarly, **chickpeas**, a staple food in children living in India, and **chestnuts** in Korea have been described as common triggers of immediate hypersensitivity in these populations. These patterns of food allergies in populations of East Asia are not commonly recognized elsewhere. It is more likely that exposure rather than genetic factors are responsible for these observations.

Fish allergens

The fish from tropical waters consumed in Asia are quite different from temperate fish. Consumption practices are also quite different. Fish is a weaning food amongst many populations in Asia. This contrasts with the Western diet, where fish is regarded as a highly allergenic food and some national guidelines on allergy prevention have recommended the avoidance of fish till the age of three. There is an impression that fish allergy in Asia is less common than in the Western world but this has not been substantiated by systemic study. Hence, the allergenicity of tropical fish is comparable with cod. The reason(s) that fish allergy is not highly prevalent in tropical Asia, despite high consumption and exposure, in early life is not obvious.

Peanut allergy

To date, there have been no published reports on population-based prevalence studies on peanut allergy in Asia, but the impression amongst clinicians practicing in Asia is that it is still uncommon, although increasing. In Singapore, a peanut allergy survey showed that the prevalence of peanut allergy was 0.3%, or about a third of those reported in Western populations. The notion that peanut allergy is not as prevalent in Asia is also substantiated by hospital-based studies on anaphylaxis. Studies from Singapore have shown that severe peanut allergy resulting in anaphylaxis was very uncommon. These data are similar to those from Thailand and Hong Kong where no cases of peanut allergy were recorded. This apparent low prevalence rate of peanut allergy in Asian populations is not likely due to lack of exposure, but more likely due to immune tolerance.

Crustacean shellfish allergy

In contrast to the low prevalence of peanut and fish allergy, crustacean shellfish appears to be an important cause of food allergy in Asia (see Chapter 2 on Epidemiology). In terms of severity, hospital-based studies on anaphylaxis show that crustacean shellfish are one of the most important food triggers in Singapore, Thailand, and Hong Kong. Interestingly, this phenomenon appears to be reversed in Western populations with less severe crustacean shellfish allergy in comparison to peanut or fish allergy. Only a few cases of crustacean shellfish-induced anaphylaxis were reported in hospital-based surveys in children in the UK and Italy, and children and adults in Australia. Instead, peanut-triggered anaphylaxis predominates in these populations.

Like fish, crustacean shellfish is a major component of the East Asian diet. However, unlike fish allergy, this increased exposure may explain the high prevalence of shellfish allergy in this region. Since exposure to fish and peanuts has not resulted in high prevalence of allergy to these food allergens in Asia, it is tempting to speculate an alternative hypothesis for the high prevalence of shellfish allergy. **The high prevalence of inhalant dust mite and cockroach allergies** in tropical and subtropical Asia may contribute to cross-reacting allergens through the allergen tropomyosin (cfr. OAS).

This hypothesis is supported by the correlation of sensitization to shrimp (Fig. 8) and cockroach allergens in Singapore children, as well as population studies on unexposed Jews who observed Kosher dietary rules, which showed that sensitization to shrimps was related to cross-reacting tropomyosin allergens in house dust mites.

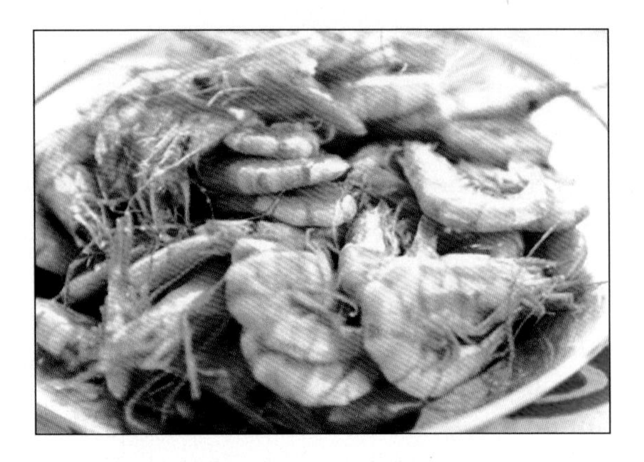

Fig 8. Prawn. The high prevalence of inhalant dust mite and cockroach allergies in tropical and subtropical Asia may contribute to the high prevalence of prawn allergy, through cross reacting with tropomyosin, which is present is house dust mites and is seafood.

Diagnosis of food allergy

A) Medical history and physical examination

The evaluation of FA must begin with a carefully taken and focused medical history and physical examination. The true value of a medical history is largely dependent on the parent's (or child's) recollection of symptoms and the examiner's ability to differentiate disorders provoked by FA and other disorders. The history may be directly useful in diagnosing FA in acute events (such as acute anaphylaxis or acute urticaria). However, problems arise when the reaction is delayed (such as in some non-IgE-mediated reactions), or occurs after several foods are ingested. An example of this is that in children with eczema, less than 50% of the reported food allergies (suspected by parents) could be substantiated by provocation tests. Moreover, if reactions occur less than two or three times weekly, keeping a food diary is cost-effective and may suggest an offending agent.

Several pieces of information are important to establish that a food allergic reaction occurred:

1. Identification of the food that provoked the reaction

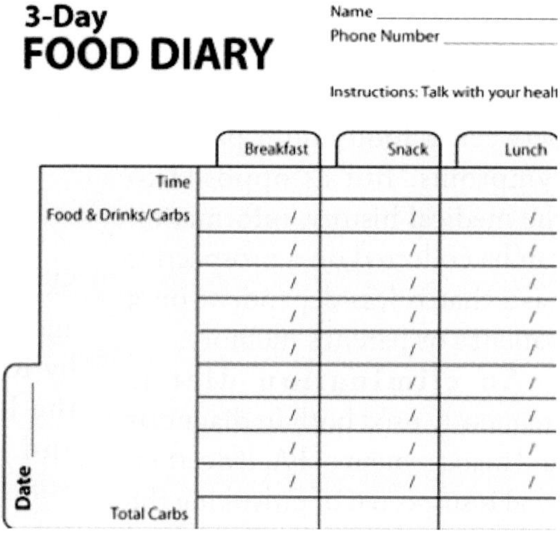

3-Day
FOOD DIARY

Name ______________
Phone Number ______________

Instructions: Talk with your healt

	Breakfast	Snack	Lunch
Time			
Food & Drinks/Carbs	/	/	/
	/	/	/
	/	/	/
	/	/	/
	/	/	/
	/	/	/
	/	/	/
	/	/	/
	/	/	/
Total Carbs			

Date ______

Fig. 9 Food diary. A diet diary can be utilized as an adjunct to the medical history, in an attempt trying to identify food is responsible for the induction of allergic symptoms.

2. The quantity of the food ingested (FA can occur after minimal amounts have been ingested)
3. The length of time between ingestion and development of symptoms (FA usually within minutes)
4. A detailed description of all the symptoms
5. If similar symptoms developed on other occasions when the food was eaten
6. If other factors are necessary (e.g. some types of FA occur preferentially after exercise)
7. The length of time since the last reaction

A diet diary (Fig. 9) has been frequently utilized as an adjunct to the medical history. Parents (or children) are asked to keep a chronological record of all foods ingested over a specified period of time and to record any symptom experienced in the child during this time. The diary can then be reviewed to determine if there is any relationship between the foods ingested and the symptoms experienced. However, uncommonly this method will detect an unrecognized association between a food and a patient's symptoms. But as opposed to the medical history, information can be collected on a prospective basis that is less dependent on a patient's or parent's memory.

An elimination diet is frequently used both in diagnosis and management of FA. If a certain food is suspected of provoking the FA, it is completely eliminated from the diet. The success of an elimination diet depends on several factors, including the correct identification of the allergen(s) involved, the ability of the patient to maintain a diet completely free of all forms of the possible offending allergen, and the assumption that other factors will not provoke similar symptoms during the study period. The likelihood of all these conditions being met is very low. Therefore, elimination diets are **rarely diagnostic** of FA, particularly in chronic disorders such as eczema. Moreover, it is very difficult to avoid food totally, as sensitization can also occur through touching or smelling of food and in infants who are totally breast fed, mother's milk can contain traces of food that the mother took (and traces of food can be sufficient to induce FA).

B) Skin prick testing and determination of specific IgE (RAST or CAP test)

Skin prick testing (SPT) (Fig. 10) and IgE determination in the blood by RAST or CAP only evaluate the IgE-mediated mechanisms and give no information on non-IgE-mediated food allergic reactions (see Chapter 11 on diagnostic tests). Usually, SPT is highly reproductive and often is utilized to screen patients for suspected Ig-E-mediated FA.

For SPT, a drop of the food extracts and appropriate control SPT (i.e. histamine as positive control and saline as negative control) are applied on the skin and the skin is gently lifted up in the drop using a small needle (prick or puncture technique). A food allergen eliciting a wheal reaction (i.e. a swelling, and not an erythema of redness of the skin) of at least 3 mm greater than the negative control is considered positive, and anything else is considered negative. However, there are two important remarks on SPT. First, a positive SPT to food indicates **a possibility** that the child has symptomatic reactivity to that specific food but is not a proof (in general

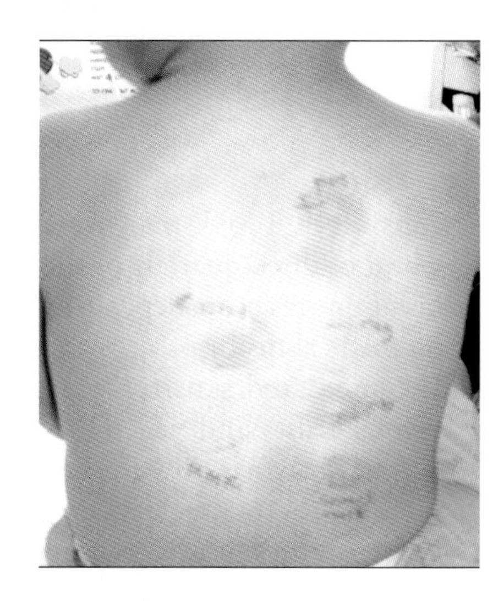

Fig. 10 Skin prick test. Skin prick testing with food only identifies the IgE-mediated food allergic reactions. However, other mechanisms can be involved in food allergy which are not detected by a positive SPT.

the positive predictive accuracy seems to be less than 50%). It means that the child has specific IgE in the blood, but this can also be found in healthy children. Second, a negative SPT confirms the absence of an IgE-mediated reaction (overall negative predictive accuracy is greater than 95%), but does not mean that the food cannot induce non-IgE-mediated reactions. Furthermore, both these remarks are only justified if appropriately standardized and good quality food extracts are utilized.

The SPT should be considered an excellent means of excluding IgE-mediated FA, but is only suggestive of the presence of clinical FA. There are minor exceptions to the general statement:

1. A positive SPT to a food ingested in isolation that provokes a serious systemic anaphylactic reaction may be considered diagnostic.
2. Children less than one year of age may have IgE-mediated FA without a positive SPT, or with minimal SPT positivity, and children less than two years of age may have smaller wheals. Usually, in young children a positive SPT is

considered a SPT that has a wheal of three-quarters of the histamine reaction, dependent on medical history.

3. IgE-mediated sensitivity to several fruits and vegetables (apples, bananas, kiwi, pears, melons, carrots, celery, etc) is frequently not detected with commercial reagents, presumably secondary to the liability of the responsible allergen in the food.

An intradermal test (injection of the allergen in the skin) is a more sensitive tool than the SPT, but is far less specific when compared to oral provocation tests, and results in a large number of **false positive results**. Furthermore, there are no studies on the sensitivity and specificity of an intradermal test in children, and it is even assumed that healthy children easily can show positive intradermal tests. In one study, no patient who had a negative SPT but a positive intradermal test to a specific food had a positive oral challenge to that food.

In addition, intradermal skin testing increases the risk of inducing a systemic reaction compared to SPT, and **should not be used in children**.

Determination of specific IgE (by the RAST or CAP method) in the blood is often used to screen for IgE-mediated FA. In general, these measurements performed in high quality laboratories provide information similar to SPT, although it seems from a number of studies that SPT is more sensitive, especially in young children. A comparison of SPT and specific IgE determination is shown in Table 3.

Table 3 Comparison between SPT and Specific IgE Determination

SPT	IgE
Sensitive (young children)	less sensitive than SPT
less specific than IgE	specific
cheap	expensive
immediate results	wait for results (according to lab)
need normal skin	for all patients
antihistamines suppress SPT	no effect of any medication
not very painful	painful
patient (and parents) can see the results	patient has to be informed by doctor

A contra-indication for a DBPCFC is a history of an obvious severe reaction to a specific food, as the challenge might induce severe reactions (example: a clear history of anaphylactic shock due to peanuts or seafood).

C) The double-blind placebo-controlled food challenge

The double-blind placebo-controlled food challenge (DBPCFC) is **the golden standard** to diagnosing adverse reactions to food, including FA.

Moreover, it is the only test to diagnose non-IgE-mediated FA, as all other tests for non-IgE-mediated FA lack sensitivity and specificity. The DBPCFC has been utilized successfully by many investigators in both children and adults. The foods to be tested are based upon history and/or SPT (or specific IgE) results. This test is the best means of controlling for the variability of chronic disorders (such as eczema) any potential temporal effects, and acute exacerbations secondary to reducing or discontinuing medications. Particularly psychogenic factors and observer bias are eliminated. The use of native fresh food for challenge is the most reliable way, although these foods need to be administered blindly, usually through a gastric tube. Alternatively, lyophilized foods (in capsules) can be administered, but sometimes the patient receives insufficient challenge material to provoke a reaction (especially in cases of non-IgE-mediated FA) or the lyophilization of the food antigens has altered the allergic potency of relevant allergens (e.g. fish).

D) Practical approach to diagnosing food allergy

The diagnosis of FA is a complex process utilizing a careful history, physical examination, SPT (or specific IgE determination), appropriate exclusion diet, and if necessary, a DBPCFC. Any other test has no value in the diagnosis. These tests include: food-specific IgG or IgG4 (commonly advised and very expensive), determination of food-antigen-complexes in the blood, and other blood tests assessing the immune system. Moreover, intradermal tests or intracutaneous tests with allergen have never been shown to be of value in diagnosing FA.

It is very important that the medical care provider makes an unequivocal diagnosis of FA. Nowadays, still too many children are labeled "food allergic" based on non-scientific criteria or suspicion. If these practices continue, over one-quarter of the population will continue to alter their eating habits, which is based on the misconception of FA, and which may induce other problems such as stigmatization, social isolation (children not allowed to attend birthday parties) and even worse, unnecessary malnutrition caused by extensive and useless diets.

Prognosis of food allergy: persist or grow out?

FA in young children is usually a favorable dynamic process in terms of long-term prognosis, as most youngsters will grow out of their FA (Fig. 11). This is mainly the case for IgE-mediated allergy for cow's milk, soy, and egg. Usually, infants grow out of a cow's milk or soy allergy by the age of two, and most of them grow out of an allergy to hen's egg by the age of four. This is also the case for non-IgE-mediated allergies of infancy. However, recent studies on **severe** allergy to cow's milk and hen's egg have shown less favorable results. Children with a severe allergy to these foods might have persistent symptoms till puberty and it was shown that those children with additional allergies and high concentrations of IgE in the blood are the ones who tended to have persistent allergy to cow's milk or eggs. The slow rate of achieving tolerance to food reported in these recent studies is alarming, but the studies emphasize that most of the children became tolerant, and reappraisal is therefore crucial, even into teenage years.

Allergies to other foods may

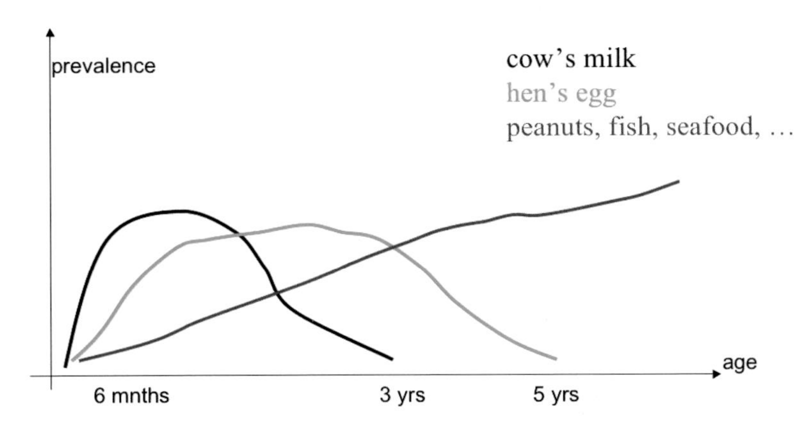

Fig. 11 Prognosis of food allergy. Every food has its own story. Some food allergies persist (fish, seafood, peanut), while other are only present for a short period.

have a persistent character. Studies have shown that FA to peanuts (80%), tree nuts, seafood, and fish can persist for a life time and that most children will not grow out of this type of FA. In adults the prognosis of a FA is even less favorable.

Whereas symptomatic FA is very specific in most patients, i.e. they do not react to more than one member of a botanical family or animal species, this is not the case in other patients, particular in pollen-related food allergy (i.e. OAS). Here, cross-reactions can even occur between phylogenetically distantly related species such as birch and kiwi or soy. Therefore, usually due to this high variety of reactions, OAS persists during adulthood. Moreover, certain factors place some individuals at increased risk for more severe or persistent reactions to food:

(1) A history of a previous severe anaphylactic reaction
(2) History of asthma, especially of poor controlled asthma
(3) Allergy to peanuts, nuts, fish, and seafood
(4) Patients on medications such as beta-blockers or ACE-inhibitors (usually in adults)
(5) Possibly being female

Treatment of food allergy

If a food is identified, the only proven therapy is the strict elimination of the food from the child's diet. However, avoidance of foods is very difficult, as contact may occur because the food is hidden in commercially prepared foods or contact may also occur through smelling. Various case reports were published of patients experiencing severe reaction by smelling peanuts (in airplanes) or fish. Therefore, it is important to continue research on active treatment of food allergy, focusing on the induction of tolerance to foods (i.e. switch of the immune system from Th2-type to Th1-type immune reactions) and on effective treatment of severe reactions.

- Various studies are ongoing on different types of immunotherapy to foods, including studies on sublingual immunotherapy (SLIT) with foods, such as peanuts. Nowadays, however, it is still too early to recommend these treatments, but in the near future effective desensitization programs might become available for those children suffering from severe FA.
- Several medications have been used in an attempt to protect children with FA. Among them are oral cromolyn, antihistamines, ketotifen, corticosteroids, and prostaglandin synthetase inhibitors. Some of these medications do modify FA symptoms in a therapeutic approach, but overall they have minimal efficacy or unacceptable side effects, especially when used long-term. However, **the use of epinephrine** is vitally crucial in acute anaphylaxis, and the importance of prompt administration of epinephrine when symptoms of systemic reactions to foods develop cannot be overemphasized. In these cases, Epipen (0.3 mg) and Epipen Jr. (0.15 mg) should be given intramuscularly immediately in a dose of 0.01 mg/kg (see also Chapter 10 on severe allergic reactions and on anaphylaxis).

Role of patient-parent education

Patient and parent education and support are essential for food allergic children. In particular, parents and older children who are prone to severe food allergic reactions must be informed in a direct but sympathetic way that these reactions are potentially fatal. In addition, when eating away from home (in schools or restaurants), food-sensitive children should feel comfortable to request information about the contents of prepared foods. Schools should also be equipped to treat anaphylaxis in allergic students (which has already been recommended by the American Academy of Pediatrics Committee of School Health in USA). Children older than seven can usually be taught to inject themselves with epinephrine, and for younger children, parents and caregivers should be appropriately instructed. Physicians must be willing to explain, and with the parents, help instruct school personnel about these issues. In the home, the elimination of foods that can cause FA in children should be considered, or if this is not practical, warning stickers should be placed on foods with the offending food allergens. A variety of support groups, including parent groups of children with FA, can help provide information, advocacy, and education.

In Singapore, information on FA can be obtained from Food Allergy Singapore (FAS). This is a non-profit volunteer operated support group, providing services for those parents and children dealing with food allergy issues as well as for anyone interested in this mission. The website is: www.foodallergysingapore.org. Similar groups of parents of children with FA exist in other countries, such as China (Shanghai and Hong Kong).

The "I CAN!" program in Singapore

"I CAN!" stands for Children's Asthma and allergy Network. It is a national program from The University Children's Medical Institute at National University of Singapore, in which holistic care is promoted for all children with asthma or allergies.

The name of the program spells the word "CAN," which signifies the ability of every child with asthma and/or allergies to participate in all activities and lead a normal lifestyle while using the least medication necessary. It reaffirms a positive outlook to the condition(s) and reminds us that all children with asthma or allergies CAN do all things

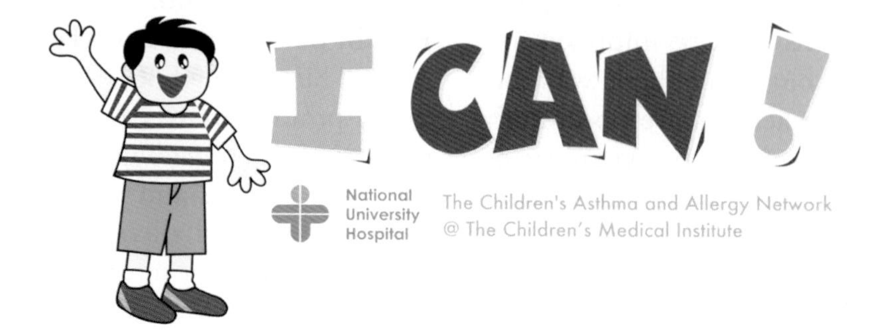

like any other child of his/her age. "I CAN!" is dedicated to the holistic care of children with asthma and allergies, encouraging close cooperation and direct communication between patients, parents, doctors, and nurses. "I CAN!" focuses on the education of patients and parents by organizing public symposia and workshops, and distributing educational materials on asthma and allergies. Scientific updates are conveyed through workshops and medical bulletins for the primary healthcare team (general practitioners, polyclinics).

Services of "I CAN!":

In-patient services

All patients hospitalized with asthma and allergy-related conditions are seen by a team of asthma and allergy specialists at the University Children's Medical Institute. All patients are thoroughly evaluated and their management optimized. The "I CAN"-team also reviews the patient and reinforces asthma education and counseling, including inhaler technique evaluation and allergen and trigger avoidance measures.

Out-patient services

Outpatients are seen at the Children's Asthma or Allergy Clinics, and when the condition is stabilized, they are encouraged to have their routine follow-up by the "I CAN!" partners

Acute facilities at the children's emergency service

Acute visits can be seen at the Children's Emergency at National University Hospital.

The program has launched a wide range of educational print materials on asthma and allergies, which are available for patients and families as well as for primary healthcare partners. These print materials are designed specially for simple reading, stimulating interest, and increasing understanding on the care and management of children with asthma and allergies. Some of the print materials that are available in this program include: asthma information booklets, asthma diaries, asthma and allergy action plans (for acute situations), education brochures, device technique cards, and newsletters.

For more info: **www.ican.com.sg**

9 Drug Allergy

A large number and type of adverse reactions to medications have been described as being responsible for substantial morbidity, even mortality. Among the adverse reactions to drugs, drug allergy (DA) constitutes a major problem with potentially fatal outcomes.

Drugs are always given because there is something wrong.
Drugs are not given to healthy subjects.
Therefore, is it sometimes difficult to distinguish drug allergy (DA) from the underlying disease, as a number of diseases can mimic DA.
Therefore, DA is a very difficult problems, and sometimes it is Impossible to find out whether the symptoms are induced by the drug or whether the symptoms are induced by the underlying disease...

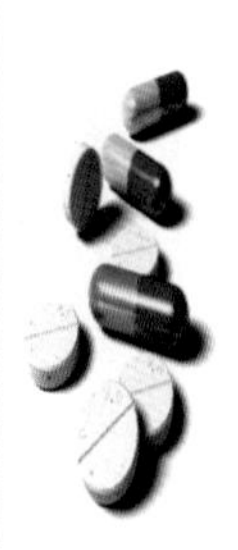

Fig. 1 A philosophical approach to DA.

Definitions and classification

An adverse drug reaction (ADR) is an undesirable and unanticipated response independent of the intended purpose of the drug. Drug allergy (DA) is an adverse drug reaction **involving the immune system**, occurring unpredictably in an otherwise normal individual.

Fear of recurrent allergic reactions often leads to avoidance of the drug of choice. Therefore, any measure in avoiding or minimizing the drug can have a major impact on the efficiency of patient care. DA is a very complex issue, because of the atypical clinical presentations in most of these patients, and the number of unknown underlying mechanisms (except IgE-mediated drug allergy), which have resulted in inadequate diagnostic tests for non-IgE mediated DA. Additionally, there is a lack of specific treatment available, other than avoidance. When evaluating a child with suspected DA, the entire spectrum of adverse reactions must be kept in mind because symptoms of many types of reaction may be similar, although the underlying mechanisms differ. Furthermore,

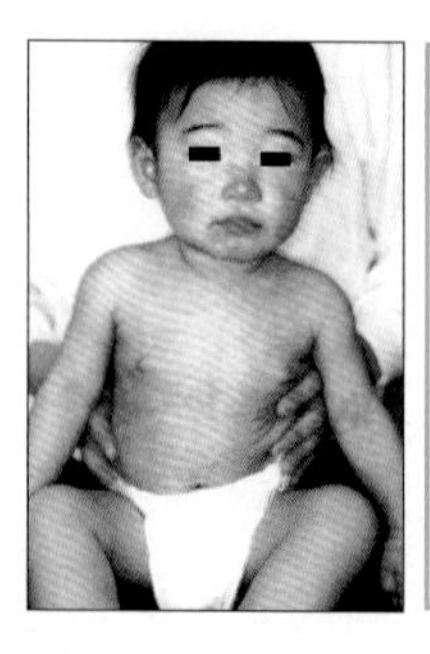

Exanthema subitum is a very common viral illness in young children, caused by a herpes virus (HV 6 and 7). Usually these children present with high fever during 3 days, and no other symptoms. On day 4, the fever drops and a rash will appear. During the first days of the illness these children are often prescribes antibiotics. As a consequence of this, the rash is often consider as a drug allergy, and these children are sometimes wrongly labeled as being drug allergic.

Fig. 2 A young child with exanthema subitum, being often mislabeled as drug allergic.

a number of viral infections, such as exanthema subitum (Fig. 2), can cause symptoms that resemble DA, and these children are often incorrectly labeled as being allergic to the drug (usually an antibiotic or paracetamol) that was prescribed during the disease.

Classification of adverse reactions to drugs

ADR can be divided in two groups: **predictable reactions** and **unpredictable reactions.**

Predictable reactions are based on the pharmacology of the drug and can occur in all individuals. These reactions include toxic reactions, side effects, drug interactions, and secondary effects.

Unpredictable reactions to drugs only occur in certain susceptible individuals. These reactions include drug intolerance, idiosyncratic reactions, DA, and anaphylactoid reactions (i.e. reactions that resemble anaphylaxis). The term DA usually refers to the IgE-mediated reaction, activating mast cells or basophiles with the release of histamine and other mediators. However, DA can also be caused by non-IgE mediated mechanisms involving the immune system, and is comparable to food allergy.

Epidemiology

Data of population-based studies on ADRs or DA, especially in large groups of non-selected children, is not available. However, from literature it seems that DA is more common in adults than in children.

In studies on hospitalized adult patients from the USA, the overall incidence of serious ADRs is estimated to be around 7%, with an incidence of 0.3% of fatal reactions. When both serious and non-serious ADRs are considered together, the percentage increases to **15%** in hospitalized adult patients.

In a retrospective study in children less than five years of age at the Children's Medical Institute, Department of Paediatrics at NUH, from 1997-2002, about **1%** of admitted children had a suspected DA. Within this group, 30% were allergic to penicillin. A subgroup of these patients underwent allergy testing and it was found that only 13% of them had a true drug allergy. Drug allergy was more common in males and there were no cases of anaphylaxis to the drugs described. The most common allergies to drugs are mentioned in Table 1.

Table 1 Drugs that are frequently associated with Adverse Drug Reactions

1. Antibiotics (especially beta-lactam antibiotics) (> 40% of all DA)
2. Sulfonamides (trimethoprim-sulfamethoxazole)
3. Insulin
4. Immunoglobulines, vaccines, antiserum
5. Local anesthetics
6. Aspirin and non-steroidal anti-inflammatory drugs (NSAIDs)
7. Paracetamol
8. Anticonvulsants

In a recent population study in Singapore using a questionnaire, our group found a prevalence of ADR of 5.4% in Singaporean children, aged seven to 16 years, with 56.7% of cases reporting

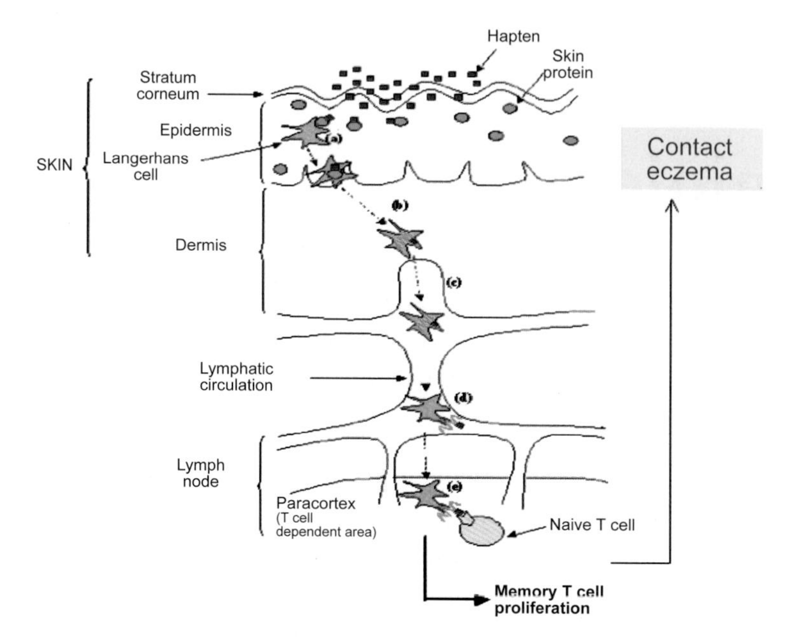

Fig. 3 Haptenation through the skin is involved in certain types of contact dermatitis (or contact eczema).

to have experienced an ADR to beta-lactam antibiotics. Of the ADRs, 60% reported dermal manifestations and multiple drug allergies accounted for 3.8%. Only 6.9% of children were referred for further diagnostic testing.

Mechanisms of allergic reactions to drugs

Except for insulin (to treat diabetes) and immunoglobulines, the molecular weight of most drugs is too low (lower than 1000) to elicit an allergic immune response (cfr. allergic immune responses are induced by proteins). However, small molecular weight drugs or their metabolites can provoke immune reactions by acting as **haptens:** they bind to the body proteins, thereby transforming them into allergens (which will be recognized by the body as foreign proteins). This process is called **haptenation** (Fig. 3).

Drugs such as **penicillin** directly bind to macromolecules on cell surfaces and in plasma to form hapten-carrier complexes. Other drugs are non-reactive with macromolecules in their native state. They are converted into reactive intermediates (i.e. metabolites) during metabolism in the liver or elsewhere by specific enzymes, such as cytochrome P_{450}-associated enzymes. The enzymes induce intracellular haptenation of proteins, which are secreted as multivalent complexes and are processed by antigen presenting cells and presented to T-lymphocytes. An example of this pathway to immunogenicity is the acetylation and oxidation metabolism of **sulfonamides** to yield the predominant N^4-sulfonamidoyl hapten.

Several factors have been identified that influence the expression of immune reactions to drugs. These factors may be related to the drug, the host, or the concurrent diseases or therapies. An overview of these influencing factors is shown in Table 2.

Table 2 Factors Influencing the Development of Drug Reactions.

Treatment-Related Factors	Patient-Related Factors
Nature of the drug or drug metabolite	**Gender and age** Higher in women and at the extremes of age.
Cross-sensitization	**Constitutional and genetic factors** Other allergic diseases and a positive family history of atopy do NOT increase the risk of DA
Route of drug administration Frequency: topical (on the skin) > IV[a] > IM[b] > oral	**Prior drug reactions** An increased risk to develop DA to new drugs
Degree and duration of exposure Large doses and frequent courses, rather than prolonged continuous treatment are more likely to induce IgE-mediated reactions. A sustained high blood level is more likely to induce a IgG-mediated reaction, such as hemolytic anemia caused by penicillin.	**Concurrent medical illness** Increased risk to develop rashes after ampicillin in EBV[c] infections and trimethoprim-sulfamethoxazole in HIV+ patients

[a] IV = intra-venous
[b] IM = Intra-muscular
[c] EBV = Ebstein-Barr virus

Certain drugs are more likely to be associated with adverse reactions than others. **Antibiotics of the beta-lactam group, such as penicillin or ampicillin**, are the commonest cause of DA and are responsible for 42% to 53% of all reported reactions. Studies indicate that patients who are allergic to one drug are not only at increased risk of reacting to another drug of the same class, but also are more likely to develop an allergic reaction to drugs of other classes. The mechanisms of this multiple drug allergy are not clear. It may be caused by an innate propensity of some individuals to develop an immune response to haptens irrespective of drug classes.

Clinical spectrum of DA

Adverse reactions to drugs often occur in a patient who suffer from an underlying pathology. The signs and symptoms are often non-specific. The fact that the patient is usually concurrently suffering from an underlying pathology (i.e. otherwise there was no reason to administer any medication) makes the diagnosis extremely difficult, and sometimes impossible, in certain situations. Many children suffering from viral-induced fever (i.e. children with common cold or pharyngitis) will develop a rash due to the underlying viral infection (more than 100 different viruses are known to be able to induce viral rashes in children, e.g. **exanthema subitum**). If a drug is taken just before the rash starts, this drug will often be implicated as the cause of the rash. This leads to the "incorrect" label of drug allergy in these patients, although no hard evidence exists on the diagnosis of a specific drug allergy.

Therefore, the diagnosis of a drug allergy on clinical grounds in patients with an underlying illness remains extremely difficult and even impossible in a number of cases. In actual fact, to make an accurate clinical diagnosis of "drug allergy", the drug should be administered to a *healthy* person. If a reaction occurs, its reproducibility should be evaluated by repeated administrations under standard conditions (drug challenge). No

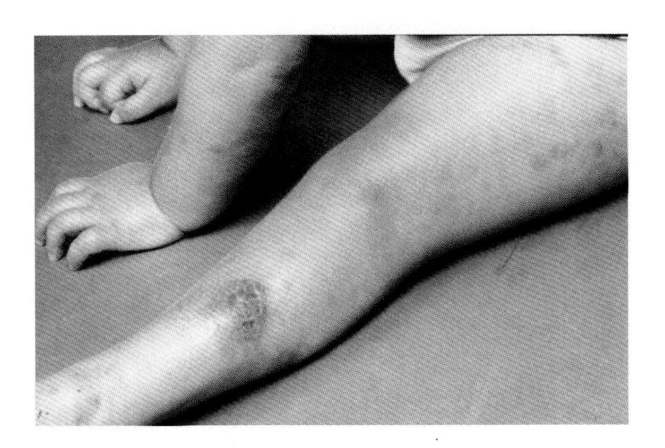

Fig. 4 Fixed drug eruption (courtesy of Prof. Lynette Sheck).

further investigations are needed except in a minority of patients experiencing severe symptoms after the administration of a specific drug (e.g. anaphylactic reactions after IV penicillin). However, most children and adults are labeled as being drug-allergic solely on clinical grounds. This practice has dangerous consequences as it may lead to situations where life-saving drugs are withheld. Therefore, the confirmation of the diagnosis of drug allergy by specific testing is recommended.

a. Severe adverse cutaneous reactions to drugs

Lesions recur in the same area when the offending **drug** is given.

The skin is the most common site of ADR, including DA. Lesions caused by drugs are usually urticaria with angioedema. Other types that have been described include vasculitis (can present as painful skin bleedings), fixed drug eruptions (Fig. 4) (lesions recur in the same area when the offending drug is given), or pustulosis (Fig. 5) (resembling skin infection).

Although the prevalence of acute severe cutaneous ADR is low, these reactions can affect any child who takes medications and can result in death or disability. Prompt differentiation of severe cutaneous ADR from less severe reactions may be difficult. Rapid recognition of severe reactions is essential and immediate

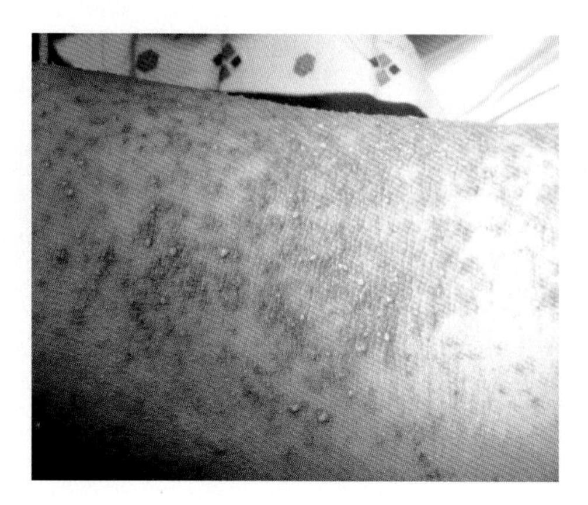

Fig. 5 Acute generalized erythematous pustulosis.

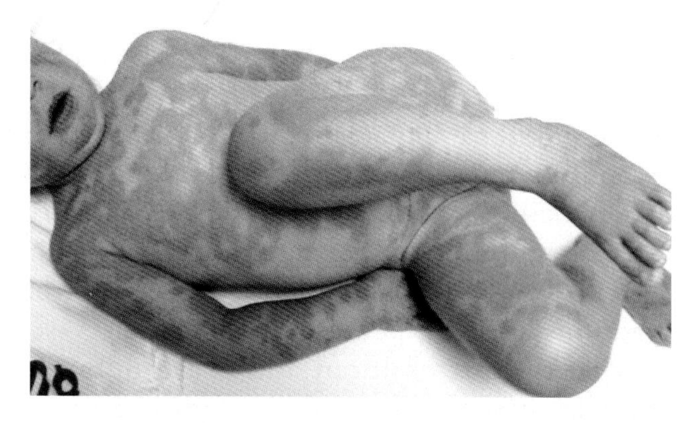

Fig. 6 Severe urticaria after administration of amoxicillin. Severe urticaria in a baby as a consequence of an allergy to amoxicillin (courtesy of Prof. Peter Smith, Australia).

withdrawal of the offending drug is often the most important action to minimize morbidity.

When an ADR is suspected, the presence of urticaria (see Fig. 6), blisters, mucosal involvement, facial edema, ulcers, palpable or extensive purpura (i.e. vasculitis), fever, or lymphadenopathy (i.e. swollen lymph nodes) almost always necessitates discontinuation of the drug. The most common severe ADRs involving the skin are listed in Table 3.

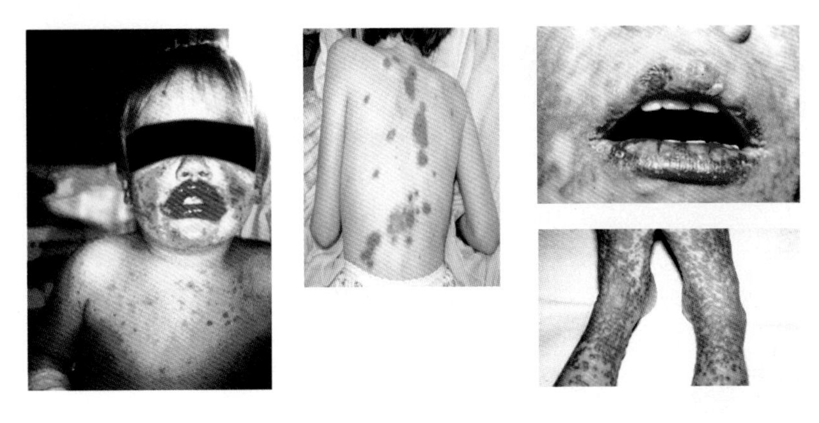

Fig. 7 Steven–Johnson syndrome induced by sulfonamides.

Table 3 Severe Adverse Skin Reactions to Drugs

Severe cutaneous drug reactions	Drugs that are most commonly involved
Stevens-Johnson syndrome (Fig. 7) Toxic epidermal necrolysis (Lyell syndrome)	trimethoprim-sulfamethoxazole sulfadoxine-pyrimethamine (Fansidar) carbamazepine hydantoins barbiturates ... and more than 100 other drugs...
Hypersensitivity syndrome (also: The anticonvulsant hypersensitivity syndrome)	antiepileptic agents - phenytoin - carbamazepine - phenobarbital allopurinol gold salts dapsone others...
Vasculitis and serum sickness	quinolones (vasculitis) amoxy-clavulate (vasculitis) cefaclor (serum sickness) minocycline (serum sickness) others...
Anticoagulant-induced skin necrosis	warfarin (in protein C deficiency)
Angioedema	penicillins NSAIDS radiocontrast media ACE inhibitors (captopril) others...

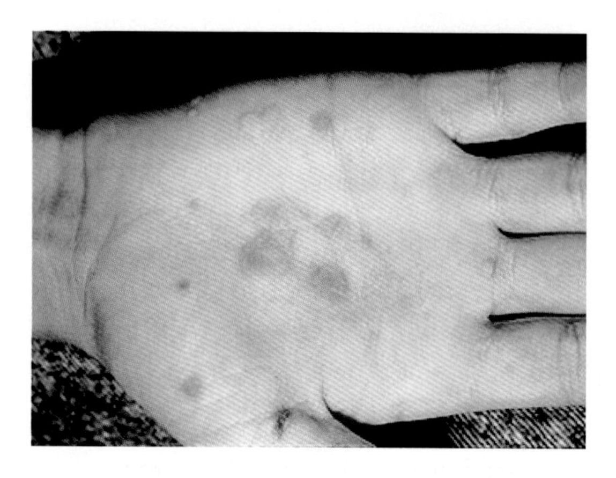

Fig. 8 Erythema multiforme major is usually not caused by drugs, but by infections (herpes simplex, Mycoplasma pneumoniae, EBV, varicella, mumps and coxsachie virus.

— **Stevens-Johnson syndrome and toxic epidermal necrolysis (Lyell)** are two severe and related mucocutaneous disorders (involving skin and mucosa) with high rates of morbidity and mortality. Stevens-Johnson syndrome is also frequently used as a synonym for **erythema multiforme major** (Fig. 8), resulting in confusion. However, it is now accepted that the two are different conditions that are usually clinically distinguishable. Children with erythema multiforme major have typical target lesions, predominantly on the extremities.

Erythema multiforme major is seldom caused by DA and usually occurs after infections, especially after herpes simplex and Mycoplasma, and has a benign course. Children with widely distributed purpuric macula and blisters and prominent involvement of the trunk and face are likely to have Stevens-Johnson syndrome, which is usually drug-induced (Table 4).

Table 4 Severe Adverse Skin Reactions Presenting as Blistering of the Skin

Table : Diagnosis	Mucosal Lesions	Typical Skin Lesions
Stevens-Johnson syndrome	Often	Small blisters on dusky purpuric macula or atypical targets, rare areas of confluence. Detachment of <10% of skin
Toxic epidermal necrolysis	Often	Lesions like SJS, but confluent erythema and large sheets of necrotic epidermis
Erythema multiforme major	Absent	Target lesions on extremities

Children suffering from Stevens-Johnson syndrome have fever, stomatitis, severe ocular involvement (conjunctivitis, and other), and a disseminated cutaneous eruption (dark-red spots, sometimes with a necrotic center). Lyell syndrome or toxic epidermal necrolysis refers to an extensive loss of epidermis due to necrosis, which leaves the skin surface looking scaled. Patients may present with Stevens-Johnson syndrome that evolves to toxic epidermal necrolysis. Although precise diagnostic boundaries between the two disorders have not been established, cases with limited areas of epidermal detachment (<10%) are usually labeled Stevens-Johnson syndrome, and those with extensive detachment as toxic epidermal necrolysis. In both disorders, involvement of the trachea, bronchi, or gastrointestinal tract may occur. Complications include massive fluid losses, infection (sepsis), and respiratory problems. A skin biopsy may help to confirm the diagnosis and exclude other diseases. Differential diagnosis includes the staphylococcal scaled skin syndrome and skin disorders involving desquamation, exfoliation, and blistering. Treatment is symptomatic and usage of corticosteroids has shown higher morbidity and mortality.

— **The Hypersensitivity Syndrome** (or anticonvulsant hypersensitivity syndrome) refers to a specific severe reaction made up by a morbilliform rash, fever, hepatitis, arthralgias, lymphadenopathy, or blood abnormalities, occurring two to six weeks after the drug is first used. Treatment with corticosteroids has been advocated, but controlled studies are lacking.

b. Severe adverse respiratory reactions to drugs

A specific type of pulmonary hypersensitivity reaction has been described as the **Löffler syndrome** or drug-induced pulmonary eosinophilia (i.e. accumulation of eosinophils in the lungs). The syndrome consists of blood eosinophilia and lung involvement, made up by transient consolidation zones that consist of eosinophilic infiltrates. The original description of the Löffler syndrome listed parasitic infection as its most common cause. However, other parasitic infections and acute hypersensitivity reactions to drugs are included as etiologies for pulmonary eosinophilia. The Löffler syndrome is considered a benign self-limiting disease without significant morbidity. Symptoms usually subside within three to four weeks or shortly after the offending medications are withdrawn in drug-induced pulmonary eosinophilia. Cough is the most common symptom among symptomatic patients. It is usually dry and unproductive, but it may be associated with production of small amounts of sputum. The Löffler syndrome has been described in all age groups, including newborns. The drug most frequently associated with the Löffler syndrome is **minocycline**, a tetracycline that is used for treating acne. Symptomatic treatment of the Löffler syndrome is the administration of high doses of corticosteroids.

- Drugs that have been described as causing the Löffler syndrome are:

- Antimicrobials – **minocycline**, dapsone, ethambutol, isoniazid, nitrofurantoin, penicillins, tetracyclines
- Anticonvulsants - carbamazepines, phenytoin, valproic acid
- Anti-inflammatory drugs and immunomodulators - aspirin, azathioprine, beclomethasone, cromolyn, gold, methotrexate, naproxen
- Other agents - bleomycin, captopril, chlorpromazine, granulocyte-macrophage colony-stimulating factor, imipramine, methylphenidate, sulfasalazine, sulfonamides

Diagnosis of drug allergy

The identification of a drug responsible for a suspected allergic reaction depends largely on history. The features of the reaction often give a clue as to whether the symptoms were caused by a drug reaction rather than by the underlying disease for which the drug was prescribed. Knowledge of all drugs that the patient has taken is important because some drugs are known to have a propensity for causing allergic reactions. Agents that have been used for long, continuous periods of time before the onset of a reaction are less likely to be implicated than agents recently introduced or reintroduced. The temporal relationship between the institution of drug therapy and the onset of the reaction is important. In individuals sensitized to a drug from prior exposure, IgE-mediated reactions typically occur within one hour of administration of the drug. Allergic contact dermatitis generally has a latency period of two to three days, and serum sickness has a latency period of about one week. In contrast, in individuals not sensitized to a drug by prior exposure, an IgE-mediated reaction generally occurs seven to 10 days into the course of treatment.

Although diagnostic tests for DA are limited, several tests do exist and may be useful. For some drugs, *in vivo* or *in vitro* tests can be done to help diagnose DA. These tests include the identification of drug-specific IgE antibodies, drug-specific T-lymphocytes, or detection of mediators from activated cells. The main limitation of these tests is the lack of availability of relevant drug antigens, and for some cases, the lack of clinical correlation. Moreover, because of the poor understanding and identification of the haptenic determinants of most drugs, **the diagnostic tests for DA are limited**.

Only for IgE-mediated reactions, including drug anaphylaxis, appropriate testing is available. As for other IgE-mediated reactions, two types of testing can be carried out: 1) the determination of serum specific IgE, and 2) skin prick testing (SPT) with the drug. Importantly, both tests can only diagnose drug allergies that are IgE-mediated. Unfortunately, there are no reliable tests for drug allergies due to other mechanisms. However, except for severe cutaneous reaction, it is usually only the IgE-mediated reactions that are

A provocation test with a drug should only be performed in a hospital under strict medical supervision.

Provocation tests should never be performed in patients with a history of a severe adverse drug reaction!

potentially life-threatening (i.e. anaphylactic shock). If these tests are positive, the diagnosis of drug allergy is very likely. No further tests should be done and the drug should be avoided. In exceptional circumstances, desensitisation procedures to a very limited number of drugs can be carried out.

If the history is compatible with DA, and if the reaction was not consistent with an IgE-mediated event or did not involve serious organ damage, a challenge (provocation testing) may be considered. Provocation testing, administrating increasing amounts of the drug, should be performed under strict medical supervision in an in-patient setting. Provocation testing should only be performed in children with negative SPT and never be performed in patients who have experienced severe ADR (i.e. Stevens-Johnson syndrome and others). In the following table (Table 5), the risks and disadvantages of provocation tests with medications are summed up:

Table 5 Risks and Disadvantages of Drug Provocation Tests

- potentially dangerous
- readout might be difficult (subjective symptoms)
- does not clarify the underlying mechanisms
- reactions are not completely typical
- false-negative results can occur
- false-positive results can occur
- co-factors that are essential for the clinical symptoms might be absent
- does not indicate mere sensitization, which may become positive under certain circumstances

In the following text of this chapter, a number of drug allergic reactions will be covered in more detail, because these reactions are important in children and because early and correct recognition may prevent morbidity of DA.

Penicillin and other beta-lactam antibiotics

Antibiotics are the commonest cause of DA in children. Of the antibiotics, beta-lactams are the commonest offenders, responsible for more than 40% of all DA reactions. The group includes the penicillins, the cephalosporines, the carbapenams, and the monolactams (see figure below).

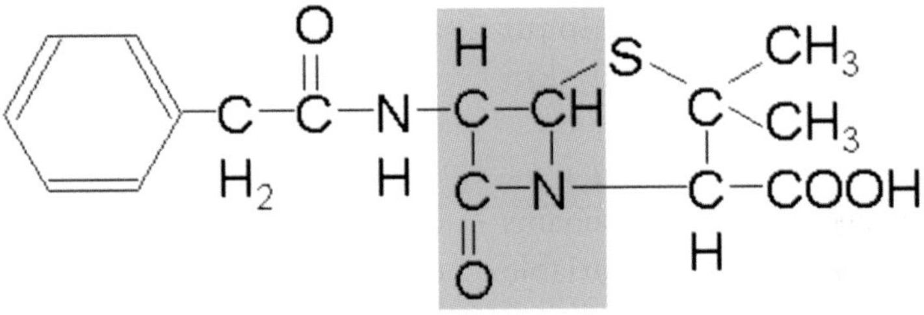

The beta-lactams can cause different types of DA, including: IgE-mediated reactions, IgG-mediated hemolytic anemia, immune complex-mediated serum sickness, and a T-cell-mediated contact dermatitis. The most common and serious reaction is **the IgE-mediated hypersensitivity reaction**. The reaction may be localized to the skin, presenting only as urticaria and angioedema, or may be anaphylactic and potentially fatal. Estimates of the incidence of hypersensitivity reactions range from 1% to 10% of patients receiving penicillin.

Penicillin is a well-studied model of haptenation. The beta-lactam ring of penicillin spontaneously opens under physiologic conditions, forming the penicilloyl group. The penicilloyl group is called ***the major determinant***, because approximately 95% of the penicillin molecules that irreversibly combine with proteins form allergens (also called penicilloyl moieties). Penicillin is also degraded to form other antigenic determinants, such as the penicillinate and penicillamine, which are formed in smaller quantities and called *minor determinants*. IgE-antibodies to the minor determinants usually cause anaphylactic reactions, while IgE to the major determinant usually induce urticarial skin reactions.

The penicillins, cephalosporines, and carbapenams share an appreciable but variable immunologic cross-reactivity. Cross-reactivity among penicillins is virtually complete. Therefore, if a patient reports an allergy to penicillin, allergy to all beta-lactams should be assumed. One exception is a late-occurring ampicillin induced skin rash during Epstein-Barr virus infections (i.e. infectious mononucleosis). Immunologic cross-reactivity between penicillin and first generation cephalosporines is high, often reported to be as high as 50%. Cross-reactivity between penicillin and second- and third-generation cephalosporines is lower: reported to be 10% or less. Carbapenams, like cephalosporines, also contain the beta-lactam ring and cross-react with penicillin. However, monolactams do not contain the beta-lactam ring and appear to lack cross-reactivity with penicillin. Sometimes, patients with penicillin allergy produce the IgE antibody to the side chain of the drug and not to the beta-lactam ring. For example, amoxicillin and cefradroxil contain the same side chain and cross-react. The monolactams, aztreonam, and third-generation cephalosporin, ceftazidime, contain the same side chain. Piperacillin and cephapyrizone also contain an identical side chain. These drug pairs therefore may potentially cross-react via side-chain reactivity rather than via beta-lactam reactivity. Independent anaphylaxis to cefazolin without cross-reactivity to other beta-lactam antibiotics has also been reported.

When DA to penicillin is suspected, SPT is the first choice investigation.

The major determinant conjugated to a poly-lysine carrier to form penicilloyl-polylysine is commercially available for skin testing. Ideally, testing to the minor determinants should also be done. However, minor determinant products are labile and are not commercially available. Determining the specific IgE to penicilloyl is another option in diagnosing IgE-mediated allergy to penicillin.

SPT and oral provocation testing (only in patients who did not experience a severe reaction to penicillin) are advocated by most investigators. Physician-diagnosed DA to penicillin (and amoxicillin and cephalosporines) based only on history and physical examination may lead to over-diagnosis. Overestimation rates of 66% have been reported if SPT and provocation testing are not performed. On the other hand, a negative SPT to penicillin does not exclude the risk for an immediate allergic reaction. In one study, a negative SPT with positive provocation test was found in 49/89 (55%) of the patients with an immediate reaction to penicillin. Specific allergy to the side-chains of penicillin may be responsible for this phenomenon. However, in other studies it was shown that penicillin can be safely administered to patients who had negative SPTs but a history of penicillin allergy. Furthermore, it has been shown that skin test reactivity can disappear or decrease with increasing intervals between the allergic reaction and the SPT. It was found that after five years, SPTs become negative in 50% of penicillin sensitive patients, while all patients with amoxicillin allergy had negative SPTs after five years. These results suggest that allergy to penicillin is not **always a lifetime persisting event**, and that a substantial number of patients can lose their allergy after three to five years.

Treatment of penicillin allergy is complete avoidance of the drug. However, if the beta-lactam antibiotic is necessary for the treatment (example: to treat a severe infection, such as meningitis), then the patient can be desensitized to the drug. This can be done by either IV or oral route, dependent on the clinical situation. Desensitization is done in a setting where close monitoring and resuscitative measures are readily available, as in an intensive care unit.

Sulfonamides

Trimethoprim-sulfamethoxazole has been increasingly used to treat and to prevent Pneumocystis carinii infections in HIV-infected patients. Since then, an increasing number of adverse reactions have been reported. The incidence of adverse reactions to trimethoprim-sulfamethoxazole in hospitalized patients is 3% to 6%. However, in HIV-positive patients the incidence is about 10 times higher. The diagnosis of sulfonamide allergy is mainly based on suggestive history. Because of the importance of sulfonamide antibiotics in HIV-patients, protocols to desensitize have been developed, but desensitization can only be considered in those patients whose reactions were minor, such as in those with dermatitis or urticaria. Patients with life-threatening skin reactions such as Stevens Johnson syndrome or toxic epidermal necrolysis (Lyell syndrome), should **not** be desensitized because re-exposure to the same drug carries a substantial risk of mortality.

Insulin

Allergic reactions to insulin in children with diabetes are uncommon, but can be either localized to the site of injection or systemic. **Local reactions** (i.e. erythema, burning, swelling, and pruritus at the site of injection) are IgE mediated, can have a late-phase reaction, and usually occur within the first two to four weeks of starting insulin, and disappear within the two to four weeks of continued treatment and without any intervention.

Systemic reactions to insulin are rare, with a reported incidence of 0.1% to 0.2%, and have decreased since the introduction of human insulin. These reactions typically occur after interruption of insulin therapy. If the reaction was severe, insulin SPT followed by desensitization is necessary. However, a positive SPT alone is not diagnostic because about 40% of diabetic patients taking insulin develop insulin-specific IgE without clinical symptoms. In patients with a suggestive history and a positive skin test, and who are not in any emergency, desensitization over several days can be done, according to existing, validated protocols.

Biological agents

Biologic agents, such as antiserum, intravenous immunoglobulin (IVIG), and some vaccines, are complete proteins and do not need haptenation to induce DA. Allergic reactions to these agents can occur, and heterologous antisera are very potent allergens. Antisera in common clinical use are anti-thymocyte globulin and antisera to rabies, snake, and spider venom. Before using these materials, it is recommended to perform SPT. Skin test positive patients need to be desensitized.

Anaphylactic reactions to IVIG are rare, but can occur in patients with a selective IgA-deficiency or in patients with common variable immunodeficiency who have anti-IgA antibodies developed prior to immunoglobulin infusions. In these patients, IVIG free of IgA should be used.

The measles-mumps-rubella (MMR) vaccine is produced in chicken-egg embryo. Trace amounts of egg proteins can be present in these vaccines, but ovalbumine (the major allergen of hen's egg) seems to be absent in MMR. Controlled studies have shown that such anti-egg reactions are extremely rare. The MMR vaccine usually can be administered safely in a single dose to children with egg allergy. Reactions to the MMR vaccine, previously attributed to egg hypersensitivity, have been shown to be due to IgE antibody formation against porcine or bovine gelatin present in the vaccine. The risk to develop an allergic reaction to **influenza vaccine** is higher in children with egg allergy, and it is recommended to perform a SPT with the vaccine in those children before administrating the vaccine.

Local anesthetics

Local anesthetic agents are relatively good sensitizers when applied topically, but antibody-mediated allergic reactions are extremely rare, especially in children. However, anaphylaxis after local administration of lidocaine in children has been described. Allergic mechanisms are often incorrectly entertained to explain adverse events, due to a response to intravenously

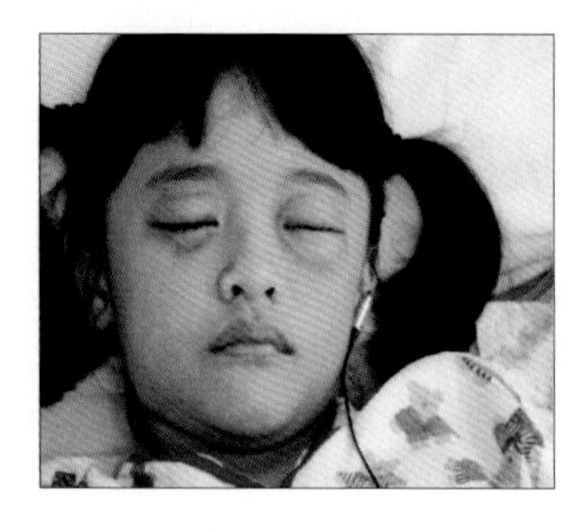
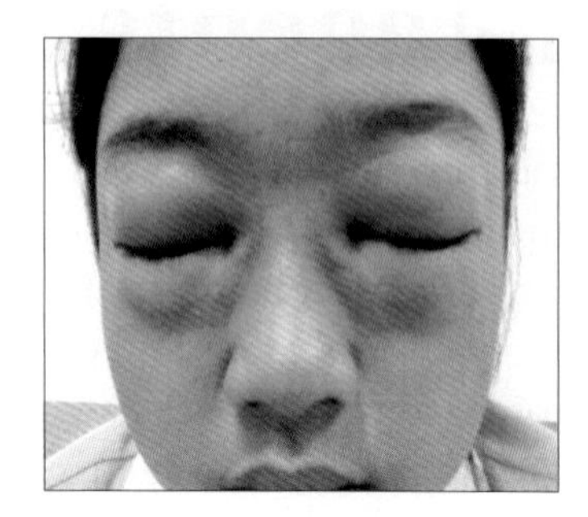

Fig. 9 An ADR to NSAIDS (ibuprofen, aspirin, etc.) usually presents as swollen eyes in children. Sometimes acute respiratory problems (asthmatic symptoms) can also occur (courtesy of Prof. Lynette Sheck).

absorbed anesthetic causing constriction of blood vessels, or a vasovagal response, anxiety or hyperventilation reaction. These responses to local anesthetics, particularly in dentistry, are a frequent cause for allergy consultations. Most alarming for patients and dentists alike are episodes of vasovagal syncope, which can mimic anaphylaxis. Because rare IgE responses to local anesthetics are reported (more in adults than in children), the goal of management is to identify the very rare patients who are truly allergic by a safe testing and challenge protocol.

Aspirin and other non-steroidal anti-inflammatory drugs (NSAIDs)

Aspirin and other NSAIDs (Table 6) can cause two types of unpredictable reactions: skin reactions manifesting as urticaria and angioedema, and respiratory tract reactions manifesting as asthma, rhinitis, nasal polyps, and sinusitis. Reactions are much more common in adults than in children (Fig. 9). The underlying mechanisms of these reactions are still incompletely understood.

Table 6 NSAIDS that Cross-react with Aspirin

Enolic acids
Piroxicam

Carboxylic acids
Acetic acids
Indomethacin, sulinac, tolmetin
Propionic acids
Ibuprofen, naproxen, fenoprofen
Fenamates
Mefenamic acid, meclofenamate
Salicylates
Aspirin, choline magnesium trisalicylate

Aspirin and other NSAIDs inhibit the cyclo-oxygenase pathway, thereby shunting arachidonic acid metabolism through the 5-lipoxygenase pathway, producing large amounts of vasoactive and bronchoconstrictive sulfidopeptide leukotrienes such as LTC4, LTD4, and LTE4. Mast cells also degranulate and release their mediators during reaction in these patients. Aspirin-sensitive individuals who manifest respiratory reactions are sensitive to all NSAIDs. However, most aspirin-sensitive patients can tolerate sodium salicylate and acetaminophen (paracetamol) at the usual dose.

The diagnosis of aspirin sensitivity is made by history and does not usually require a challenge test. For patients in whom the diagnosis is unclear and in whom a specific diagnosis is necessary, oral aspirin/NSAIDs challenges can be done, using a standardized protocol. The treatment of aspirin sensitivity is strict avoidance of aspirin and all NSAIDs. In patients for whom aspirin is absolutely essential, desensitization can be performed. Long-term aspirin desensitization has been shown to improve control of rhinosinusitis and asthma, reduce steroid requirement for asthma control, and prevent polyp re-growth. Patients with aspirin-induced urticaria and angioedema cannot be desensitized. Attempts at desensitization result in severe flare-up of the skin manifestations, which do not remit until aspirin therapy is discontinued.

Paracetamol (acetaminophen)

ADRs to paracetamol (acetaminophen) are rare and only very few clinical data are available. However, paracetamol hypersensitivity has been described in both adults and children. Underlying mechanisms are unknown, but a non-IgE mediated pathway seems likely. The presence of increased levels of serum histamine during anaphylactic reactions suggest direct degranulation of mast cells and basophils by paracetamol. Diagnosis is made by oral provocation testing. If diagnosis is based only on history, 85% of the patients are labeled false positive. Most allergic reactions to paracetamol are skin eruptions (rash, urticaria), although anaphylactic shock has been described. Children who are hypersensitive to paracetamol are usually tolerant to acetylsalicylic acid. Patients who are allergic to NSAIDs usually show good tolerability of paracetamol.

Anaphylactoid drug reactions

Anaphylactoid drug reactions are caused by direct degranulation of mast cells and basophils without activation of the IgE-IgE receptor pathway. One characteristic of anaphylactoid reactions that distinguishes them from anaphylaxis is the first-dose phenomenon. As opposed to classic IgE-mediated anaphylaxis, which requires a sensitizing dose, the first exposure to a drug can cause an anaphylactoid reaction. Examples of drugs causing anaphylactoid reactions are: radiocontrast media, vancomycin, ciprofloxacin, and opioids.

The conventional high-osmolar radiocontrast media have an osmolarity of about seven times higher than that of plasma. *In vitro* studies show that at this high osmolarity, mast cells and basophils release their mediators. The incidence of reactions to these agents is about 5% to 8% in a general population. Fatal reactions have been reported to occur in about one in 50 000 procedures. The newer low-osmolar radiocontrast media have only twice the osmolarity of plasma and appear to induce fewer reactions. The incidence of anaphylactoid reactions is reported to be about 2% with the newer agents. Once a patient has had an anaphylactoid reaction to a high-osmolar radiocontrast medium, the risk of another reaction to the same agent is as high as 30%. For these high-risk patients, pretreatment with prednisolone and diphenhydramine reduces the rates of reaction to 10%. Adding epinephrine further reduces the rate to about 7.5%.

IV vancomycin has been associated with pruritus and erythema over the upper body (i.e. the red neck or red man syndrome). The total dose of the drug and the rate of infusion influence the release of histamine and the development of signs and symptoms. The reaction can be reduced or avoided by decreasing the rate of infusion. Vancomycin can also cause a classic IgE-mediated anaphylactic reaction. In the latter case, desensitization rather than reducing the infusion rate is necessary.

Prevention and treatment

In choosing a drug, doctors should avoid drugs that are likely to cause sensitization. Drugs like heterologous antisera can induce sensitization in a large percentage of the population. Therefore, if the need arises for the use of the same type of drug again, it is advisable to choose an alternate drug with similar efficacy or to skin test the patient to rule out sensitivity. Furthermore, intermittent use of large parenteral doses of drugs (i.e. penicillin) should be avoided.

A detailed drug allergy history is valuable in preventing an allergic reaction to a drug. If a patient had an adverse reaction to a drug, that particular drug, as well as those that may cross-react should be avoided. If absolutely essential, appropriate *in vivo* or *in vitro* testing and desensitization should be performed.

There is no good treatment for drug allergy except avoidance of the drug. Desensitisation protocols for penicillin, vancomycin, and insulin have been described, but should only be considered in exceptional cases.

Most patients with drug allergy have a favorable prognosis, except in those few cases with severe

IgE-mediated allergic reaction (anaphylactic shock) and in those with severe cutaneous reactions (Stevens-Johnson syndrome). Therefore, retesting and re-provocation should be considered after withholding the drug for one to two years. For penicillin, retesting after three to five years is recommended.

Treatment of drug-induced symptoms is purely symptomatically, including the administration of epinephrine, antihistamines, corticosteroids, and beta-agonists, depending on the type and severity of the reaction. An adrenaline kit (such as Epipen) is only recommended in select patients with severe and multiple drug allergies.

Conclusion

Virtually all drugs (even corticosteroids and antihistamines) can cause ADR, including DA (for instance, the contact dermatitis by local application of the corticosteroid budesonide). Drug allergy is a very difficult issue, because of the multivariate mechanisms and clinical symptoms. Furthermore, the underlying disease for which the drug was administrated may mask, complicate, and influence the symptoms of DA. That's why most patients (especially children) are incorrectly labeled as being drug-allergic. Therefore, it is advisable that appropriate diagnostic testing is performed to confirm the clinical suspicion of drug allergy, especially in those children with a vague history and in cases of suspected multiple DA.

10

Severe Allergic Reactions: What Can We Do?

In this chapter, severe allergic reactions, referred to as anaphylaxis and anaphylactic shock (i.e. drop of blood pressure) are potentially life-threatening systemic allergic reactions that can affect the whole body. Anaphylaxis occurs when the immune system overreacts to an allergen. The flood of mediators and cytokines released from different cells involved in the allergic reactions (such as mast cells and basophils) during anaphylaxis makes the blood pressure drop suddenly and the airways narrow (i.e. asthmatic symptoms), causing difficulty in breathing or even unconsciousness and death (see Fig. 1). The anaphylactic response may occur within seconds or minutes of exposure to an allergen. Although anaphylaxis is the most dangerous type of allergic reaction, it is also

10

Severe Allergic Reactions: What Can We Do?

Introduction

In this chapter, severe allergic reactions, referred to as **anaphylaxis** and anaphylactic shock (i.e. drop of blood pressure), are potentially life-threatening systemic allergic reactions that can affect the whole body. Anaphylaxis occurs when the immune system severely reacts to an allergen. The flood of mediators and cytokines released from different cells involved in the allergic reaction (such as mast cells and basophils) during anaphylaxis makes the blood pressure drop suddenly and the airways narrow (i.e. asthmatic symptoms), causing difficulty in breathing or even unconsciousness and death (see Fig. 1). An anaphylactic response may occur within seconds or minutes of exposure to an allergen. Although anaphylaxis is the most dangerous type of allergic reaction, it is also

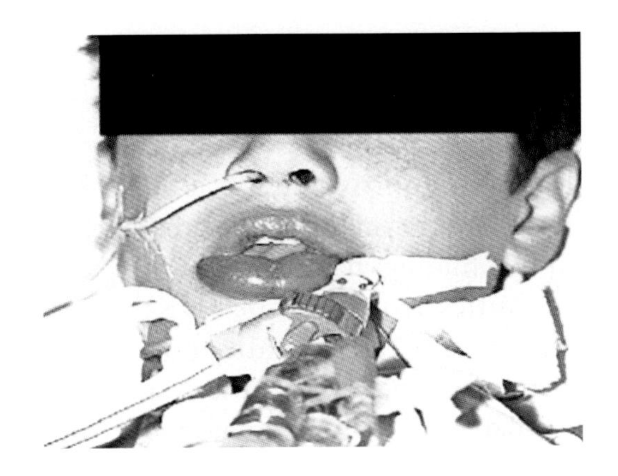

Fig. 1 Boy in anaphylactic shock. (Courtesy of Prof. Giden Lack, London).

the least common. Fortunately, patients can be instructed to respond quickly and effectively to an anaphylactic reaction by knowing the signs and symptoms and by carrying emergency medication. It is also important to instruct patients to do everything to prevent exposure to life-threatening causes of anaphylaxis allergens.

The term **anaphylaxis** is usually used for severe IgE-mediated immune responses. A second term, **non-allergic anaphylaxis,** is also in use, and describes a number of clinically identical reactions that are not immunologically mediated. The clinical diagnosis and management are, however, identical.

Epidemiology

Most of the epidemiological studies come from the USA, and only a few studies have been performed in Asia, such as in Korea, Thailand, Hong Kong, and Singapore. Food allergy is one of the major causes of anaphylaxis in children. Therefore, the prevalence of food-induced anaphylaxis varies with the dietary habits of the region. A USA-survey reported an annual occurrence of 10.8 cases per 100 000 person years, resulting in approximately 29 000 food-anaphylactic episodes each year, and approximately 2000 hospitalizations and 150 deaths. Similar findings have been found in studies from Europe (UK, France, and Italy), while food allergy was reported to cause over one-half of all severe anaphylactic episodes in Italian children treated in emergency departments.

Anaphylaxis is thought to be less common in non-Westernized countries, although it has been suggested that it is increasing in Asia. In a study from Thailand on patients admitted to Siriraj Hospital (Bangkok), it was found that the prevalence of anaphylaxis increased from 9.16 per 100 000 admitted persons in 1999 to 55.45 per 100 000 admitted persons in 2004. A study, published in 2008 from Seoul National University Hospital reported that 0.014% of admitted patients had anaphylaxis. The authors concluded that the incidence, mortality rate, and clinical features of Korean patients with anaphylaxis were similar to rates for patients from other countries. A study from Singapore on adult patients admitted with anaphylaxis concluded that the pattern of food-induced anaphylaxis differs from Caucasian populations, likely to be because of different regional dietary patterns and methods of food preparation.

Signs and symptoms

An anaphylactic reaction usually occurs in susceptible patients with a history of allergy to food, medication, or insects (e.g. wasps, bees), but can also occur in children with a negative past medical history, and in some cases the cause of the reaction remains unknown. The effects of anaphylaxis are not limited to the site of the exposure, but involve the whole body.

Development of the following signs and symptoms within minutes of exposure to an allergen is a strong indication of anaphylaxis:

- Urticaria and angioedema, with itching (usually as a first symptom)
- Constriction of the airways, inducing wheezing and a swollen tongue or throat,

which results in difficulty breathing; symptoms can start with an "itchy throat"
- Shock associated with a severe and rapid decrease in blood pressure
- Weak and rapid pulse
- Coma (i.e. decreased consciousness, including dizziness or fainting
- Flushed or pale skin (shock)
- Nausea, vomiting, or diarrhea

Symptoms originating from different sites (organs) of the body can be involved in the symptom complex of anaphylaxis. Different organs can be involved in anaphylaxis.

The most common include:

Gastro-intestinal: Abdominal pain, hyperperistalsis with faecal urgency or incontinence, nausea, vomiting, diarrhea.

Oral: Pruritus of lips, tongue and palate, edema of lips and tongue.

Respiratory: Upper airway obstruction from swelling (angioedema) of the tongue, oropharynx or larynx; bronchospasms, chest tightness, cough, wheezing; rhinitis, sneezing, congestion, runny nose.

Cutaneous: Diffuse erythema, flushing, urticaria, pruritus, angioedema.

Cardiovascular: Faintness, hypotension, arrhythmias, shock, syncope, chest pain.

Ocular: Periorbital edema, erythema, conjunctival erythema, tearing.

Genito-urinary: Uterine cramps, urinary urgency, or incontinence.

Causes and risk factors of anaphylaxis

Many allergens can cause anaphylaxis. Sometimes the cause of an anaphylactic reaction is unknown. The most common causes of anaphylaxis include:

- Medication, such as penicillin
- Foods such as peanuts, tree nuts (walnuts, pecans), milk, eggs, fish, and shellfish
- Insect stings from bees, yellow jackets, wasps, hornets, and fire ants
- Latex

In the USA, peanuts are responsible for more than 90% of fatalities caused by anaphylaxis. Data from other countries are missing. In the table below, the most common foods inducing anaphylaxis in 124 Singaporean children arriving at the emergency room are shown:

Table 1 Food Causing Acute Anaphylaxis in Singaporean Children

	% of children	mean age of the children
1. Egg and milk	11 %	0.7
2. Bird's nest	27 %	4.5
3. Chinese herbs	7 %	5.0
4. Crustacean seafood	24 %	11.0
5. Others*	30 %	7.0

*Chicken, duck, ham, fruits (banana, rambutan), cereals, gelatin, and spices

Study performed at NUS, Department of Pediatrics (published in *Allergy* (1999), **54**: 84–86).

Causes of anaphylaxis

1.`IgE-Mediated Reactions

Foods (Table 1)

In theory, any food proteins are capable of causing an anaphylactic reaction. Foods most frequently implicated in anaphylaxis are:

- Peanuts
- Tree nuts (walnut, hazelnut/filbert, cashew, pistachio nut, Brazil nut, pine nut, almond)
- Fish
- Shellfish (shrimp, crab, lobster, oyster, scallops)
- Milk (cow, goat)
- Eggs
- Seeds (cotton seed, sesame, mustard)
- Fruits, vegetables
- Bird's nest (a cause of anaphylaxis in Singapore)

Food sensitivity can be so severe that a systemic reaction can occur to particle inhalation, such as the odors of cooked fish or the opening of a package of peanuts.

A severe allergy to pollen, for example, ragweed, grass or tree pollen, can indicate that an individual may be susceptible to anaphylaxis (i.e. oral allergy syndrome).

Food-associated, exercise-induced anaphylaxis may occur when individuals exercise within two to four hours after ingesting a specific food. The individual is, however, able to exercise without symptoms, as long as the incriminated food is not consumed before exercise. The patient is likewise able to ingest the incriminated food with impunity as long as no exercise occurs for several hours after eating the food.

Antibiotics and other drugs

Penicillin, cephalosporin, and sulphonamide antibiotics

Penicillin is the most common cause of anaphylaxis. Serious reactions to penicillin occur about twice as frequently following intramuscular or intravenous administration versus oral administration, but oral penicillin administration may also induce anaphylaxis.

Muscle relaxants

Muscle relaxants, such as suxamethonium, alcuronium, and others, which are widely used in general anesthesia, account for 70-80% of all allergic reactions occurring during general anesthesia. Reactions are caused by an immediate IgE-mediated hypersensitivity reaction.

Insects

Hymenoptera venoms (bee, wasp, yellow-jacket, hornet, fire ant) contain enzymes such as phospholipases and hyaluronidases and other proteins, which can elicit an IgE antibody response.

Latex

Latex-related allergic reactions can complicate medical procedures, e.g., internal examinations, surgery, and catheterization. Medical and dental staff may develop occupational allergy through the use of latex gloves.

Foreign proteins

Examples of foreign proteins that can cause anaphylaxis are insulin, seminal proteins, and horse-derived antitoxins, the latter of which is used to neutralize venom in snake bites.

2. Cytotoxic and Immune Complex- Complement-Mediated Reactions

Whole blood, serum, plasma, fractionated serum products, immunoglobulines, dextran

Anaphylactic responses have been observed after the administration of whole blood or its products, including serum, plasma, fractionated serum products, and immunoglobulines. One of the mechanisms responsible for these reactions is the formation of antigen-antibody reactions on the red blood cell surface or from immune complexes resulting in the activation of complement. The active by-products generated by complement activation (anaphylatoxins C3a, C4a, and C5a) cause mast cell (and basophile) degranulation, mediator release and generation, and anaphylaxis. In addition, complement products may directly induce vascular permeability and contract smooth muscle. Individuals who have IgA deficiency may become sensitized to the IgA provided in blood products. Those selective IgA deficient subjects (1:500 of the general population) can develop anaphylaxis when given blood products, because of their anti-IgA antibodies (probably IgE-anti-IgA).

Cytotoxic reactions can also cause anaphylaxis via complement activation. Antibodies (IgG and IgM) against red blood cells, as occurs in a mismatched blood transfusion reaction, activate complement. This reaction causes agglutination and lysis of red blood cells, as well as perturbation of mast cells resulting in anaphylaxis.

3. Non-Immunologic Mast Cell Activators

Radiocontrast media, low-molecular weight chemicals

Mast cells may degranulate when exposed to low-molecular-weight chemicals. Hyper-osmolar iodinated contrast media may cause mast cell degranulation by activation of the complement and coagulation systems. These reactions can also occur, but much less commonly, with the newer contrast media agents.

Narcotics

Narcotics are mast cell activators capable of causing elevated plasma histamine levels and non-allergic anaphylaxis. They are most commonly observed by anesthesiologists.

4. Modulators of Arachidonic Acid Metabolism

Aspirin, ibuprofen, indomethacin, and other non-steroidal anti-inflammatory agents (NSAIDs)

IgE antibodies against aspirin and other NSAIDs have not been identified. Affected individuals tolerate choline or sodium salicylates, substances closely structurally related to aspirin but differ in that they lack the acetyl group.

5. Sulfiting Agents

Sodium and potassium sulfites, bisulfites, metabisulfites, and gaseous sulfur dioxides

These preservatives are added to foods and drinks to prevent discoloration and are also used as preservatives in some medications. Sulfites are converted in the acid environment of the stomach to SO_2 and H_2SO_3, which are then inhaled. They can produce asthma and non-allergic hypersensitivity reactions in susceptible individuals.

6. Idiopathic Causes

Exercise

Exercise alone can cause anaphylaxis as can food-induced anaphylaxis. Exercise-induced anaphylaxis can occur during the pollinating season of plants to which the individual is allergic.

Idiopathic Anaphylaxis

Flushing, tachycardia, angioedema, upper airway obstruction, urticaria, and other signs and symptoms of anaphylaxis can occur without a recognizable cause. Diagnosis is based primarily on the history and an exhaustive search for causative factors.

Risk factors

Anaphylaxis is not a common manifestation of allergy, though many people are at risk of having an anaphylactic reaction. If patients have a history of allergies or asthma, they may be at increased risk — especially if they had an anaphylactic reaction before. Future reactions may be more severe than the first.

Screening and diagnosis

The first step in the diagnosis of a past anaphylaxis is a medical history, including a detailed description of the symptoms, the treatment that was administrated, and the possible causes of the anaphylactic reaction (such as food, medication, and insect bites). If parents have experienced an episode of anaphylaxis in their child or think the child might have experienced some of the signs and symptoms associated with it, **they should be advised to see a doctor.** An evaluation typically includes questions about:

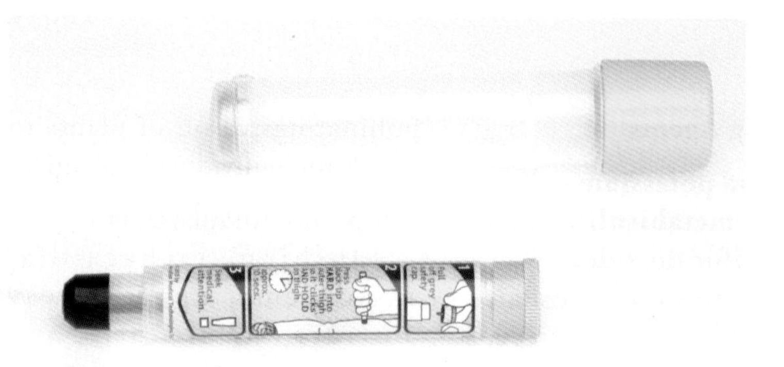

Fig. 2 The Epipen can be a life Saving treatment. Instructing and training the child and the parents is crucial of optimal usage.

- Food
- Medications
- Latex
- Insect stings

After a medical history and a physical examination that are suggestive for anaphylaxis, allergy testing should be performed without any delay (it is important to make the diagnosis as soon as possible). However, if the cause is obvious and the reaction was severe, it is not necessary to perform further allergy testing.

If a past anaphylaxis is suspected by history, the parents and child should be instructed on how to prevent future anaphylactic reactions and on how to treat it by self-administration of medication.

Parents may also be asked to keep a detailed list of the child's eating habits.

Treatment

Adrenaline (epinephrine) is the drug most commonly used to treat anaphylactic reactions. It can be self-administered with an auto-injector, such as the Epipen (Fig. 2), and Epipen Junin (children).

An auto-injector is a combined

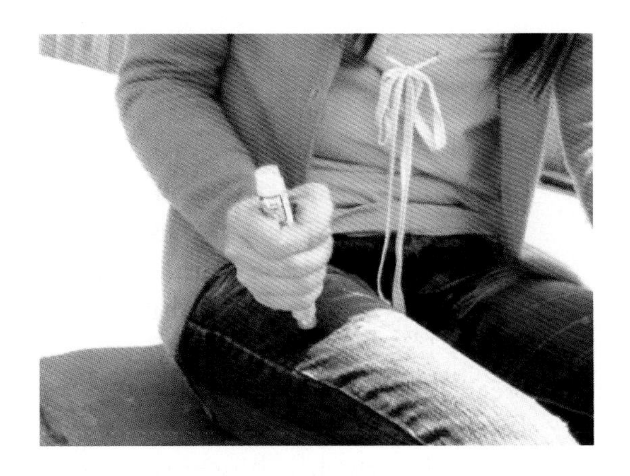

Fig. 3 Child using Epipen. Self-administration of the Epipen can be life saving.

syringe and concealed needle that injects a single dose of medication when pressed against a muscle. Usually, it is advised to inject the thigh of the child, but any muscle can be used for injection. Children with a history of anaphylaxis should be advised to carry an epinephrine (Fig. 3) auto-injector with them. **Parents and (older) children should be carefully instructed (repeatedly) on how to use the auto-injector properly.**

Also, people closest to the child (older siblings, family members, school personal) should be instructed on how to administer the drug.

In cases of anaphylaxis, and if necessary, a doctor or emergency medical team may perform cardiopulmonary resuscitation (CPR). They may also administer intravenous antihistamines and corticosteroids to reduce ongoing inflammation.

An approach to anaphylaxis is the following:

If you're with someone who has experienced anaphylaxis and shows signs of shock — pale, cool and clammy skin, weak and rapid pulse, shallow breathing, confusion, anxiety — follow these steps:

- Call 911 (Singapore 995) or seek emergency medical help immediately.

- Check to see if the person is carrying special medications to treat an allergy attack. If so, administer the medication.
- Get the person to lie down on his or her back. Elevate the feet higher than the head to keep adequate blood flow to the brain, which will prevent fainting. Keep him or her from moving unnecessarily.
- Keep the person warm and comfortable. Loosen tight clothing and cover him or her with a blanket. Don't give the person anything to drink.
- If the person is vomiting or bleeding from the mouth, place the person on his or her side to prevent choking.

If the person isn't breathing or has no pulse, perform CPR.

Emergency Treatment

For all emergencies, including anaphylaxis, the following approach is recommended worldwide, also called "ABC."

Check A = Airway

Ensure and establish a patent airway, if necessary, by repositioning the head and neck. Place the patient in a supine position and elevate the lower extremities. Patients in severe respiratory distress may be more comfortable in the sitting position.

Check B = Breathing

Assess adequacy of ventilation and provide the patient with sufficient oxygen to maintain adequate oxygen saturation. Treat bronchospasms as necessary. Equipment for endotracheal intubation should be available for immediate use in the event of respiratory failure and is indicated for respiratory failure or airway obstruction not responding immediately to supplemental oxygen and epinephrine.

Check C = Circulation

Minimize or eliminate continued exposure to the causative agent by discontinuing the infusion, as with radio-contrast media, or by placing a venous tourniquet proximal to the site of the injection or insect sting. Assess adequacy of perfusion by taking the pulse rate, blood pressure, and the capillary refill time. Establish IV access and administer an isotonic solution such as normal saline. A second IV may be established as necessary. If a vasopressor, such as dopamine, becomes necessary, the patient requires immediate transfer to an intensive care setting.

Prevention

The best way to prevent anaphylaxis is to avoid substances that are known to cause this severe reaction. Follow these steps to help ensure your well-being:

- Wear a medical alert necklace or bracelet to indicate if you have an allergy to specific drugs or other substances.
- Alert your doctor to your drug allergies before having any medical treatment. If you receive allergy shots, always wait at least 30 minutes before leaving the clinic so that you can receive immediate treatment if you have a severe reaction to the allergy shot.
- Keep a properly stocked emergency kit with prescribed medications available at all times. Your doctor can advise you on the appropriate contents. This may include an epinephrine auto-injector. Make sure your auto-injector has not expired. These medications generally last 18 months.
- If you're allergic to stinging insects, exercise caution when they're nearby. Wear long-sleeved shirts and trousers. Avoid bright colors and don't wear perfumes or colognes. Stay calm if you come in proximity to a stinging insect. Move away slowly and avoid slapping at the insect.
- Avoid wearing sandals or walking barefoot on the grass if you're allergic to insect stings.
- If you have specific food allergies, read the labels of all the foods you buy. Manufacturing processes can change, so it's important to periodically recheck the labels of foods you commonly eat. When eating out, ask about ingredients in the food, and ask about food preparation because even small amounts of the food you're allergic to can cause a serious reaction.

What can parents do if their child develops an anaphylactic reaction?

In case of anaphylaxis in their child, parents can do the following:

1. Be sure that the child is in a comfortable position and call for emergency medical help immediately or prepare to go to an emergency room nearby.
2. In the meantime, give the following medications:

All children experiencing anaphylaxis or suspected of anaphylaxis should be seen by a doctor ASAP!

- **Epinephrine (Epipen)** as soon as possible, even in mild (starting) cases of anaphylaxis. Parents should not doubt and stop the increase of the anaphylactic reaction by administrating Epipen ASAP. Better to give than not (or wait till it is too late).
- A high dose of an **oral antihistamine** might be useful (although not proven) if the child is not unconscious (if unconscious there is a risk of aspirating the syrup into the lungs). Don't use sedating antihistamines as their effect (sedation) might mask the development of shock. Only use fast-acting, non-sedating antihistamines.
- **A beta-agonist** (such as a Ventolin inhaler) if the child has respiratory symptoms

Conclusion

Fortunately, anaphylaxis is uncommon, but when occurring should be treated ASAP. Children and parents (and caregivers) should be properly instructed how to treat, especially how to administer epinephrine, using an Epipen.

11

Diagnosis and Management of Allergic Diseases

Diagnosis of allergy: allergy testing

The diagnosis of an allergic disease is largely based on the history of the patient and from clinical examination. The data can then be confirmed by allergy testing. However, in some patients further allergy testing is not even necessary, as results from the history and clinical examination are specific and sufficient to make the diagnosis.

Example: *A child developing acute urticaria within minutes of eating peanuts does not need further allergy testing because the diagnosis is obvious.*

In other patients, however, the history is less clear and the association with an underlying allergy can not be made from the history or clinical examination. This is usually the case in children who are allergic to allergens to which they are chronically exposed, such as house dust mites or pets. Allergy testing in these patients is necessary to make the diagnosis and to start specific treatment, such as allergen avoidance.

Example: *A child with monthly bronchitis, due to hypersensitivity of the airways, maintained by an underlying house dust mite allergy.*

The purpose of allergy testing is to confirm a suspected underlying allergy in a patient, using tests that have been proved to be of **scientific value**.

Unfortunately, there are now numerous non-scientifically proven diagnostic tests and treatments available, and the number of unproven tests is still increasing. Unproven allergy tests and treatments are procedures that lack scientific credibility and have not been shown to be of value. They came into being because some people became disappointed with classical medicine and were looking for better medical care, mainly because of the lack of information on allergy. Many parents still hope that their children can be cured, and they do not accept controller treatments. They do not realize that an **allergy is mainly a genetic disease** and that it is therefore impossible to cure most allergies. The only treatment that has a proven curative effect, but only in selected patients, is immunotherapy, including sublingual immunotherapy (see below). All other treatments only have a controlling effect: once the treatment is stopped, symptoms will re-occur.

Therefore, alternative medicine has become very popular among parents of allergic children, mainly because of the false promises that they make: curing the child without any long-term treatment and without the risk of side effects. Expectations of successful results from "natural" or "soft" methods without "chemicals" or from Chinese or Tibetan medicine are high. These procedures are promoted by small groups of physicians, usually because they base their practice on controversial and unproven theories, and by the manufacturers of these unorthodox tests or treatments, due to obvious commercial interests.

Till today, there is no scientific evidence that any type of alternative medicine has any diagnostic or therapeutic value in allergic children!

There have been a large number of studies on allergy testing, concluding that only a limited number of diagnostic tests are of value in diagnosing allergy. Moreover, other studies came to the conclusion that alternative allergy tests (used by different types of alternative medicine) are totally worthless (and expensive), and should never be used in diagnosing allergic diseases in children.

The diagnostic tests that have value in children are:

1. Skin prick tests (still considered as the "**golden standard**" in diagnosing allergy).
2. Determination of specific IgE in the blood.
3. Provocation tests (in which the allergen is administered to the patients, and symptoms are monitored).

In theory, the provocation test is the best test, because it highlights the ability to mimic the real life situation. However, provocation tests have a number of disadvantages, such as that **severe symptoms might be induced**. Therefore, provocation testing has a very restricted indication, and should only be performed if really necessary, and under maximum safety conditions (in a hospital, with all emergency equipment available).

In the next part of this chapter, skin prick testing will be described more extensively, including its comparison to the determination of specific IgE in the blood.

1. Skin prick testing and the determination of specific IgE

Skin prick testing

In daily practice, skin prick testing (SPT) is still considered a key diagnostic tool (i.e. the test of choice) in diagnosing allergy

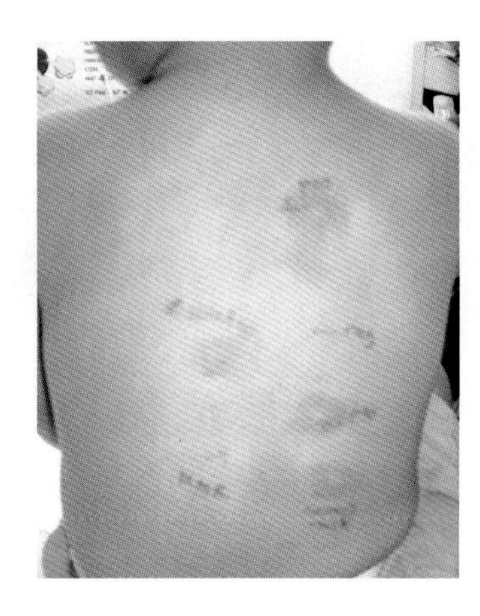

Fig. 1 Positive skin prick tests on the back of a 15-month-old child.

in children and adults (see also Chapter 8 on Food Allergy). Especially in young children (Fig. 1) and infants, SPT is more sensitive than the determination of specific IgE. SPT is not only cheap and rapid, but is also an accurate way of identifying the causative allergens. Moreover, SPT is uncomplicated, and with practice and adherence to a few simple guidelines, it is possible to get highly reproducible results. SPT is particularly useful in young children, but can also be used in selected cases for the diagnosis in food, drug, and insect allergy. In the future, more sophisticated antibody assay methodologies (such as emerging protein array technology) might become the standard in allergy diagnosing, replacing the role of SPT.

1. *Mechanisms*

SPT depends on the introduction of an allergen into the dermis (skin) resulting in an IgE-mediated response, which is characterized by an immediate wheal and flare reaction.

When the allergen is introduced into the skin on a previously sensitized individual, IgE molecules on the surface of a mast cell are bridged, and degranulation of the mast cell occurs. Preformed granules containing histamine and other mediators are released, which

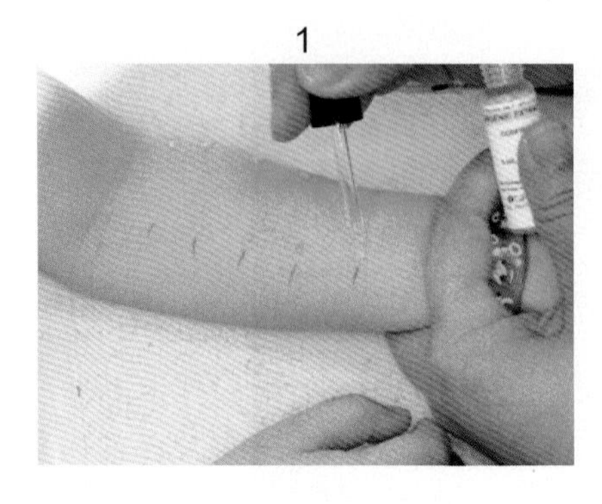

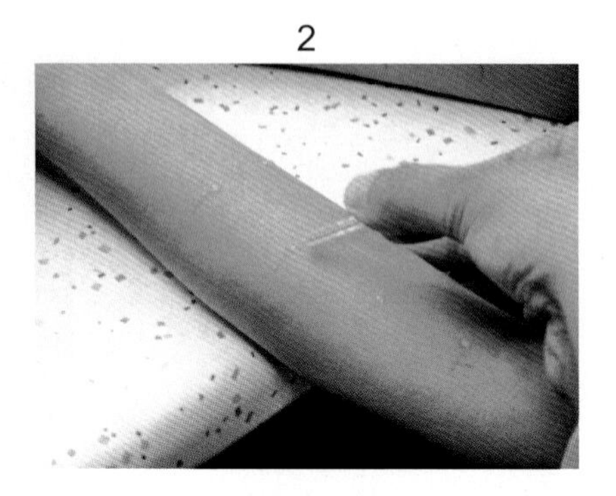

Fig. 2 Two pictures of technique (lancet in skin) of SPT. A drop of allergen is put on the skin (1) with a small needle the skin is gently lift up in the drop, (2) without causing any bleeding (cfr. prick through drop).

might induce the progressive infiltration of the dermis of eosinophils and neutrophils, which have been attracted to the site by chemotactic factors, inducing a late cutaneous response. Some agents, however, may induce mast cell histamine release by non-IgE mediated mechanisms (e.g. morphine or codeine).

2. *Technique*

SPT is best performed on the volar or inner aspect of the forearms (Fig. 2) avoiding the flexures and the wrist areas.

Under the age of three, SPT may more easily be performed on the child's back.

It is important to explain the SPT procedure to children and parents. This will lead to co-operation and a positive attitude from parents and children. The skin must be clean and free of active eczema. A grid can be marked with a pen at 2 cm intervals and a drop of the relevant allergen placed on the arm at the end of each line. The pattern follows a corresponding list of allergens used for easy identification. Standardized panels of allergens, according to age and local epidemiological data, are used in most centers.

A lancet with a 1 mm point is used to gently prick the skin through the drop, with minimal discomfort to the child. With the so-called **"prick through drop"** method it is unnecessary to scratch or lift the skin and no blood should be drawn. Reactions should occur within 10-15 minutes, after which the results can be assessed. A positive and negative control must be included in each series of tests. The negative control solution is the diluent used to preserve the allergen extract. The positive control solution is a 1 mg/ml histamine hydrochloride solution and is used to detect hyporeactivity of the skin, including suppression by medication. Another useful positive control, especially in young children, is codein, a mast cell degranulator and marker of the presence of mast cells in the skin.

3. *Interpretation of SPT results*

It is important that each clinic is consistent with respect to the method it uses to report its SPT results. In general, a wheal reaction of 3 mm greater than the negative control, with an appropriate histamine wheal reaction of 3 mm or more, is regarded as positive. In infants, a SPT reaction is positive when the wheal is at least three-quarters of the histamine reaction. Grading of SPT may be expressed in absolute values (millimeters - centimeters), or as a percentage of the positive histamine control, or may be measured as follows:

+	3 mm wheal with flare
++	3 to 5 mm wheal with flare
+++	> 5 mm wheal with flare
++++	> 5 mm wheal with flare and pseudopodia

Results may also be recorded using transparent tape over the wheal and flare and marking the size of the wheal and flare using a koki or felt tipped pen. Usually, the results for inhalant allergens are more reliable than those for foods (which can induce a number of false positive reactions, especially in children with atopic dermatitis).

In some patients a delayed skin reaction occurs about three to five hours after the skin test

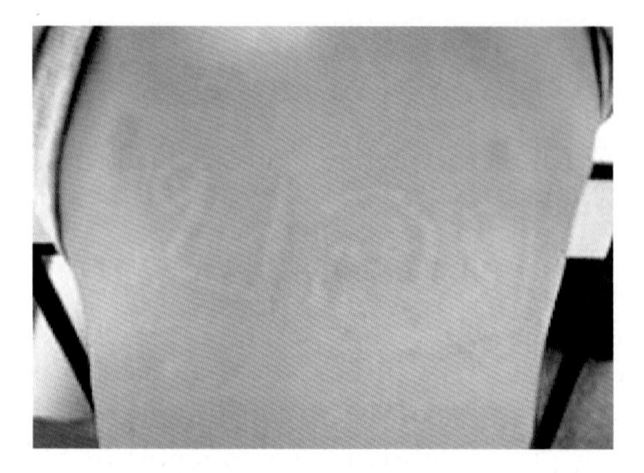

Fig. 3 Dermographism. A very sensitive skin to pressure, allowing to write on the skin by using just a little pressure.

has been performed (the so-called late cutaneous reactions), and it is important to remind all patients to look out for these.

Nowadays, devices are available to directly measure the transverse and longitudinal diameters of skin prick test wheals or flares in centimeters. More recently, a scanning method has been developed, computing the area of wheal or flare and recording the data in a computer (Prick-Film, Immunotek, Madrid, Spain).

- **Dermatographism** (Fig. 3) may occur as a result of the child's skin being excessively sensitive to friction or pressure rather than to an allergen. If the patient exhibits this reaction, then the negative control will also show a wheal and flare reaction. Any reading 3 mm larger than the negative control will then be read as positive.

Furthermore, it is important that the child is in a good clinical condition at the time of the SPT, in order to perform the test on a normally functioning immune system. Severe infections or prolonged fever may suppress the results of SPT. The influence of underlying malignancies or chemotherapy on SPT has not been assessed.

4. *Safety of SPT*

Systemic reactions are extremely rare, especially in children, but may occur if the SPT is performed in a severe unstable asthmatic patient or in a pollen-sensitive patient at the height of the pollen season. Care should also be taken when testing patients with severe food allergy (such as in children with systemic reactions to peanuts) and in patients with severe drug allergy. Therefore, it is recommended to have the following emergency resuscitative equipment available:

Injectable Adrenaline 1:1000 (Epipen)

Oxygen

Oral and injectable antihistamine (cetirizine or promethazine)

Hydrocortisone

Inhaled bronchodilator, e.g. salbutamol

However, from daily clinical practice, it can be concluded that SPT is a safe and reliable test to diagnose allergy in children (even infants) and adults.

5. *Indications for SPT*

A. To diagnose an underlying allergy in a child suffering from rhinitis, eczema, asthma, and urticaria: It is recommended to use standardized panels according to age and according to local epidemiological data on allergic diseases. In our institution in Singapore, two standardized panels to screen for allergy are in use: one for young children (under three years old) and one for older children. Allergy screening in young children is focused on food allergy, while in older children it is directed towards screening for allergy against inhaled allergens. According to specific history (i.e. food allergy, drug allergy, etc), other allergens can be added to the panel. However, other allergies are extremely uncommon, and SPT with these allergens should only be performed if the history of the child is suggestive for that type of allergy.

PANEL – YOUNG CHILDREN (< three years old)

1. **House dust mites**
2. **Cat**
3. **Cow's milk**
4. **Egg white**
5. **Soy**
6. **Others per indication (wheat, other food)**

PANEL – OLDER CHILDREN (> three years old)

1. **House dust mites**
2. **Cockroaches**
3. **Cat**
4. **Others per indication (dog, moulds, pollen, food).**

B. To diagnose venom allergy and IgE-mediated drug allergy

C. To evaluate the effect of specific allergen immunotherapy (SIT and SLIT) and to monitor its efficacy at regular intervals in selected patients.

D. To monitor changes in allergen sensitivity over a period of time (e.g. growing out of food allergy) or upon the re-emergence of symptoms.

6. *Factors influencing SPT*

- All **antihistamine containing medications,** including cough mixtures that contain antihistamines, need to be stopped prior to testing as they effectively block the wheal and flare reaction (Table 1). In general, it is recommended to stop all antihistamines for one week before SPT.

Table 1 Blocking of IgE-mediated SPT

A. Marked Blocking	
Drug	**Duration**
Clemastine	(1-10 days)
Hydroxyzine	(1-10 days)
Ketotifen	(5 days)
Chlorpheniramine	(0.5-3 days)
Promethazine	(0.5-3 days)
Cetirizine	(1-2 days)

B. Variable Blocking
Specific immunotherapy
Theophylline
Oral and injected beta agonists
Oral steroids

C. Non Blocking
Inhaled beta agonists
Cromolyn

Other conditions affecting results of SPT

1. Infants and young children may have low skin reactivity (due to low numbers of mast cells in the skin), and interpreting SPT in young children can be difficult and requires skill.
2. Severe eczema and also old eczema lesions may cause hyporeactivity of the skin, because of intensive subcutaneous scarring (thickening) of the skin.
3. Incorrect technique and loss of potency of allergy solutions due to incorrect or prolonged storage.

In conclusion, SPT is safe, simple, and cheap, with immediate reproducible results available to the clinician, the child, and the parents. In conjunction with the case history and clinical findings, SPT still remains the key diagnostic tool in childhood allergic diseases.

Determination of specific IgE

IgE is the antibody responsible for allergic reactions. Determining allergen-specific IgE in the blood of the patient is therefore of value in diagnosing the existence of an allergy. Several methods to determine IgE in serum (blood) have been developed. The old methods showed little sensitivity and specificity, but with the new methods, determination of specific IgE is highly reliable, showing good sensitivity (detection of low concentrations) and specificity (few false positive results).

Therefore, determination of **antigen-specific IgE** is a better method than the determination of total IgE to diagnose allergy, and its value is similar to skin prick testing. Nowadays, there are more than 400 characterized allergens available for *in vitro* diagnostic tests and several useful methodologies for specific IgE determination. Specific IgE results obtained with the different methods vary significantly, with absolute agreement in about 55-65% of cases. The specificity of the anti-IgE antibody used in the assay is of critical importance because any contaminant antibody can render unspecific results. On the other hand, it must be pointed out that there is a compromise between specificity and sensitivity, such that an increase in the sensitivity of a technique leads to a decrease in its specificity. One method cannot be said to be better than others; it is better to carry out the examination individually, allergen by allergen. Thus, specific IgE determination varies depending on the type of allergen. In general terms, for inhalant allergens, specificity and sensitivity of the methods are within the range of 85-95%, but these values (especially the specificity) decrease in the case of food allergens, and they are still lower when the allergen is a beta-lactam antibiotic. There is a good correlation between clinical history and specific IgE against inhalant allergens, and a lower correlation in the case of food allergens. Due to the fact that most food allergens are not standardized, the definitive diagnosis of food hypersensitivity is still achieved by means of double-blind placebo-controlled provocation tests.

The first immunometric assay, called the radioallergosorbent test (RAST), was developed in 1967. This assay was patterned after the RIST (radioimmunosorbent) assay for total IgE, except instead of coupling anti-human IgE to activated paper disks (for determining total IgE), the allergen was directly coupled to make an allergosorbent (solid-phase allergen reagent) (Fig. 4).

In one current assay (the Pharmacia CAP system), a cellulose sponge was activated and used to bind large amounts of allergens, thereby increasing the sensitivity of the test. In another clinical assay (AlaSTAT), the allergen was conjugated with biotin, and once added to the reaction mixture in solution-phase chemistry, the biotinylated allergen-IgE antibody complex was bound to a solid phase via an avidin-biotin bridge.

The different IgE antibody assays can be classified into qualitative, semiquantitative, and quantitative categories, depending on the degree to which their results accurately reflect the quantity of IgE antibody in serum. In *qualitative IgE antibody assays*, a preassigned positive threshold level is used to determine if a result is **positive** (reactive) or **negative** (non-reactive). The positive threshold is assigned by analyzing sera from non-atopic individuals with low total serum IgE levels who are known to be clinically not allergic by history and skin prick testing. Qualitative assays tend to be the least complex of the tests performed. *Semiquantitative IgE antibody assays* provide the magnitude of the response measured. The

The RAST test

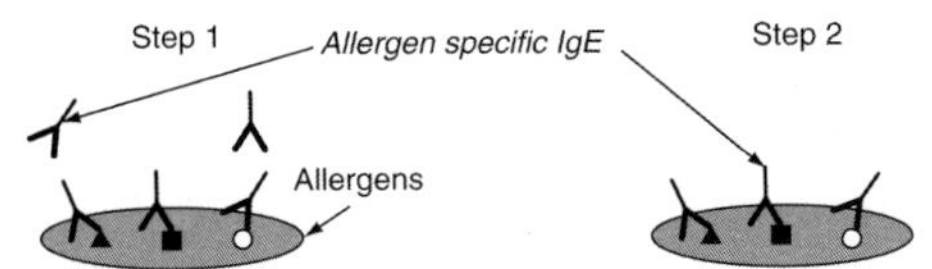

The serum sample is incubated with an allergen disc. During this step, IgE molecules with specificities for the various allergenic components bind to the allergen disc.

Proteins non-specifically bound are washed away with a buffer containing detergent. Only specifically bound IgE remains on the disc.

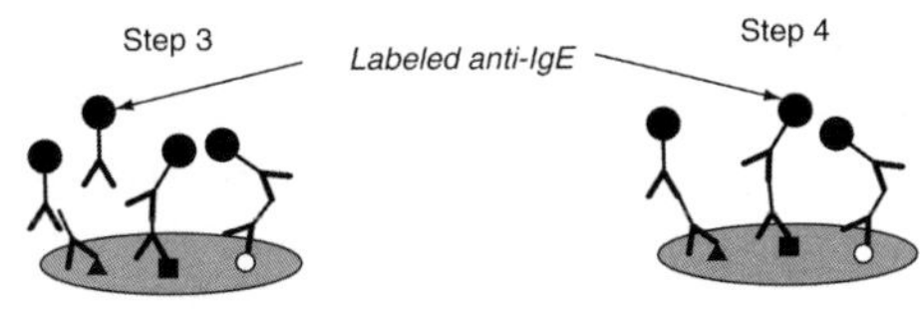

The disc is incubated with labeled anti-human IgE antibody, which binds specifically to the IgE on the disc. The amount of labeled antibody bound is directly proportional to the amount of IgE present on the disc.

Unbound antibody is washed away with buffer containing detergent.

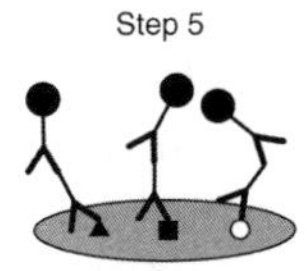

Specific IgE is quantitated either through the reaction of labeled antibody with an enzyme substrate (EIA), or by countiong radioactivity (RAST).

Fig. 4 RAST test: a test to determine specific IgE in the blood.

level of the response is related in terms of rank order, but is not directly proportional to the quantity of IgE antibody present in the test serum. *Quantitative IgE antibody assays* employ the most advanced assay calibration methods. The most widely used calibration system in commercial IgE antibody assays is a total serum IgE curve that is traceable to the WHO 75/502 IgE primary standard. For clinicians who use international units, allergen-specific IgE antibody response data are interpolated from the total serum IgE calibration curve in kIUa/L levels of allergen-specific IgE antibody. As in the total serum IgE assay, 1 IU/ml is equivalent to 2.4 ng/ml of IgE antibody.

Remark on total IgE

While specific IgE is directed against specific allergens, total IgE is the sum of all IgE present in the blood, not only against allergens, but also against micro-organisms, such as viruses or parasites. The value of determining total IgE, via RIST, in diagnosing allergy is **limited**, as it only gives an idea about the potential of the patient to produce IgE. Although many allergic patients have a raised total IgE, this can also be found in non-allergic patients, for instance, in children after viral or parasitic infections. Therefore, total IgE determination is considered a method for the screening of allergic diseases, though its actual value is controversial because normal values of total IgE do not exclude the existence of an allergic disease, and high values of total IgE are not specific of allergy on itself.

2. Non-diagnostic tests (tests that have no value in diagnosing allergy)

Unfortunately, a large number of non-scientific tests are available now, and the list is still increasing. Parents of allergic children should be aware that these tests have no value and some such tests are expensive.

Moreover, the results of these tests might lead to incorrect treatments, such as the prescription of extensive diets, which might be very troublesome (for the whole family) and harmful for the child, even leading to malnutrition. On the Internet, under "Allergy – unproven methods", one can find much data and comments from many health authorities and non-profit organizations on these tests.

The purpose of this text is to warn parents about these tests, allowing them to avoid employing these tests on their allergic children.

The most commonly used non-diagnostic tests for allergic children can be divided in two groups: tests *in vivo* (on the child) and tests *in vitro* (on the blood of the child).

- *In vivo* tests

1. Applied Kinesiology: muscle testing for allergies

The idea of this test (Fig. 5) is that every organ dysfunction is accompanied by a specific muscle weakness, which enables diseases to be diagnosed through muscle-testing procedures. The concepts of applied kinesiology do not conform to scientific data

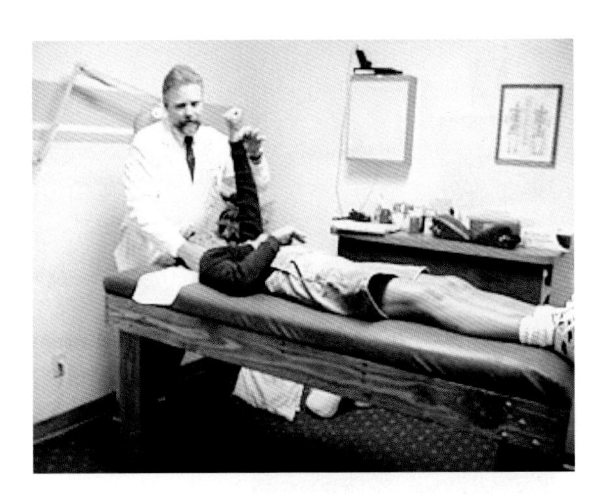

Fig. 5 Applied kinesiology is rubbish.

about the causes or treatments of diseases, and controlled studies have found no difference between the results with test substances (usually food) and with placebos. Differences between one test and another may be due to suggestibility, distraction, variations in the amount of force or leverage involved, and muscle fatigue.

2. Electrodermal skin testing, bioresonance, and dubious devices

Some physicians, neuropaths, dentists, and chiropractors use "electrodiagnostic" devices (Fig. 6) to help select the treatment they prescribe, which usually includes homeopathic products. The diagnostic procedure is most commonly referred to as Electro-acupuncture according to Voll (EAV) or Electrodermal screening (EDS), but some practitioners call it bioelectric functions diagnosis (BFD) or bio-energy regulatory technique (BER). The devices they use are simply resistance-measuring instruments, and the effectiveness or accuracy of these different techniques has not been shown.

Bioresonance is based on the belief that human beings as well as any substances in the environment, such as allergens, emit electromagnetic waves, which may be either "good" or "bad". These waves can only be measured by specific bioresonance devices, but it was shown that the devices are not capable of

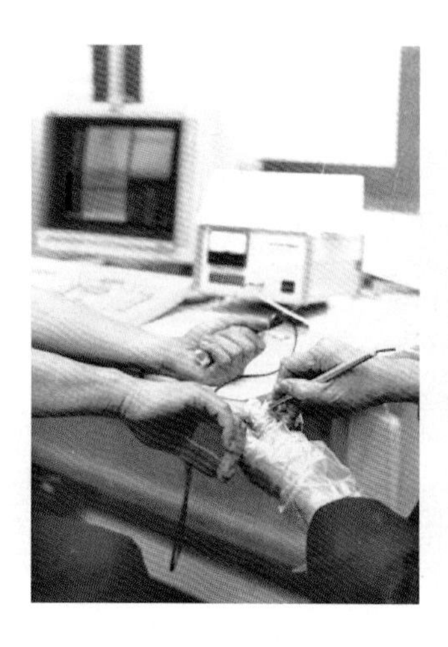

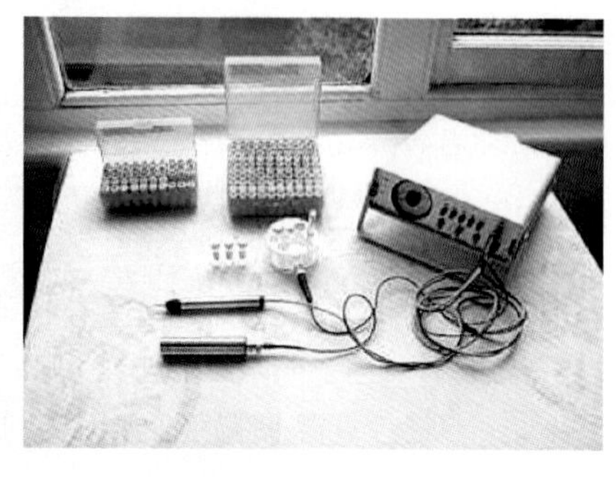

Fig. 6 Electrodermal tests have no value in diagnosing allergy.

measuring the electromagnetic waves presumed to be involved. Bioresonance therapy uses the apparatus, which is supposed to be capable of filtering the waves and sending the "rehabilitated" waves to the patient. It is claimed that the pathologic waves can be removed by that process, and the allergic disease should thereby be treated. However, controlled studies failed to show any diagnostic or therapeutic value of bioresonance in adults suffering from allergic rhinitis and in children with eczema.

In short, the tests described above are used to diagnose non-existent health problems, select inappropriate treatments, and defraud insurance companies. The practitioners who use them are either delusional, dishonest, or both. These tests should be confiscated and the practitioners who use them should be prosecuted.

- *In vitro* tests

1. Cytotoxic testing: ALCAT

The ALCAT test (TEST FOR CELLULAR RESPONSES TO FOREIGN SUBSTANCES) has been launched in several countries for diagnosing so-called "non-IgE-mediated hypersensitivities". The promotion is mainly: "for detecting adverse reactions to foods by advanced technology".

The ALCAT test is a more sophisticated version of the previous "leukocytotoxic testing", which was stopped in the USA by government actions after a negative statement of the American Academy of Allergy, Asthma and Immunology (AAAAI), concluding that cytotoxic testing is ineffective for diagnosing food or inhalant allergies.

The basic principle of the ALCAT test is measurement changes in white blood cell diameter after challenge with foods, molds, food additives, environmental chemicals, dyes, pharmaco-active agents in foods, antibiotics, and other medications *in vitro*. The blood cells are passed through a narrow channel and are measured by an electronic instrument, allowing the instantaneous counting of the number of cells in a parallel series of size, ranging from the smallest to the largest. The sizes are displayed as either cell diameter or cell volume. Using an electronic principle, histograms of the different samples are produced. According to the information brochure, the system has proven to be extremely reproducible and sensitive. In the company homepage several references are listed, mainly from papers presented at congresses or articles in non-peer reviewed journals. Therefore, it can be concluded that the ALCAT test system is relying on unproven statements that lack scientific and clinical proofs of efficacy, and is a test system that has no value in diagnosing allergic diseases in children.

2. Determinating allergen specific IgG and IgG4

Specific IgG and IgG4 (a subclass of IgG) can be found in both adults and children in many different physiological (normal) and pathological (abnormal) conditions, and their levels mainly reflect contact with allergens, and is in no way a measurement of disease. The concentrations of IgG and IgG4 drop after a period of withdrawal of specific antigens (no contact means no production of IgG and IgG4). The determination of allergen-specific IgG or IgG4 with different appropriate methods (immune precipitation, passive hemagglutination, IgG RAST/CAP, ELISA, and chemiluminescence) alone do not prove the existence of an underlying allergy, as positive tests can also be found in healthy

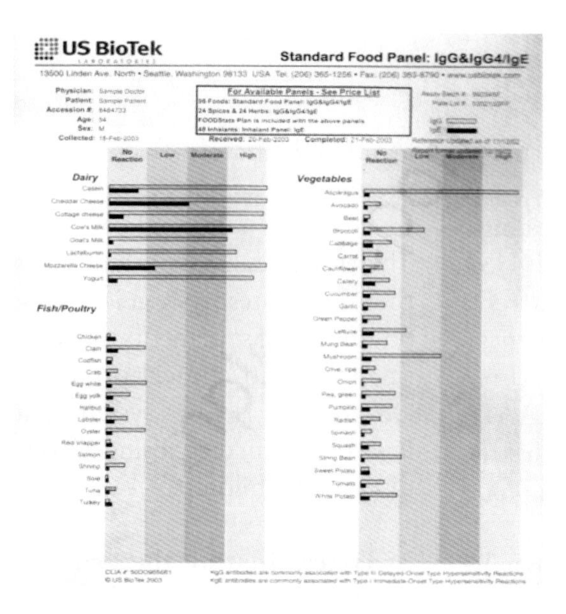

Fig. 7 IgG against allergens. Determination of IgG has no value in diagnosing allergy in children.

subjects. Furthermore, it was found that the determination of food-specific IgG failed to distinguish between subjects who responded to a double-blind placebo-controlled provocation test with food and those who did not respond after a provocation test. Taken together, there is absolutely no evidence that the determination of specific IgG or IgG4 to allergens has any value in the diagnosis of an underlying allergy.

3. The "Food Allergy Profile"

A number of alternative doctors now use the so-called *Food Allergy Profile IgE and IgG* (Fig. 7) against more than 100 foods. The results are given in color with a scale of reactivity (0+ to 3+). The patient then receives information about the results and therapy in the form of a *True Relief Guide* with instructions based on a first phase of *Elimination diet* of the IgG positive foods and on a second phase with the *Rotation Diet Schedule*. In this phase, foods that are not eliminated are allowed. After having eliminated the foods the patients were advised to avoid for a period of time determined

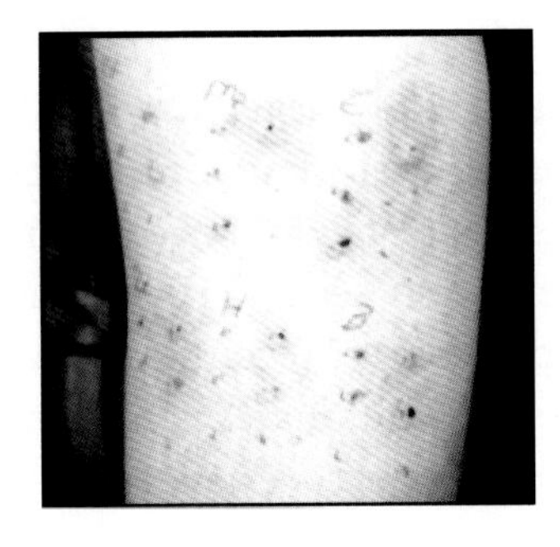

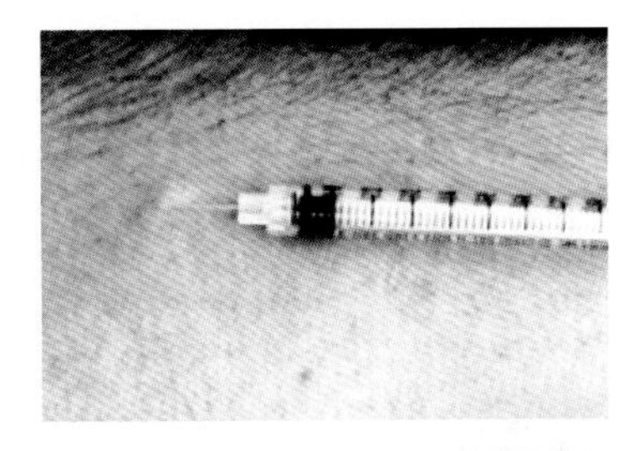

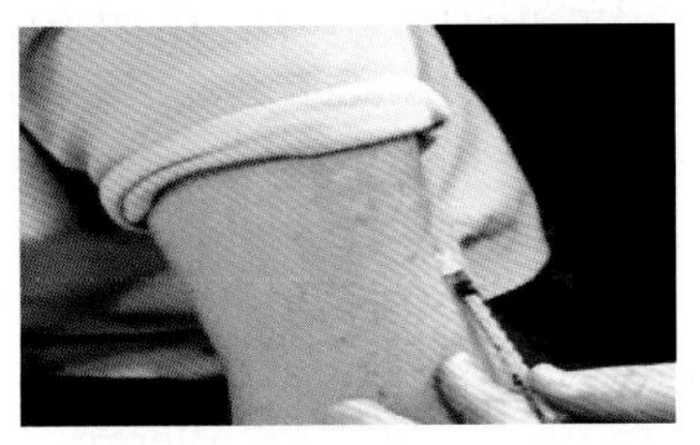

Fig. 8 Intradermal testing has no value in the diagnosis of allergy in children.

by a computer program on the basis of the results (1+, 2+, 3+) (e.g. three, six, or nine months), and having rotated other foods to prevent the development of new allergies, the foods may be reintroduced into the diet (third phase). That procedure is not economical, lacks all scientific evidence, and can be dangerous if a true IgE-mediated allergy is still present after the avoidance phase. Obviously, such a sophisticated guide is impressive for patients and parents, and together with the charisma of their health care providers (?) using these mystic elimination, rotation and reintroduction diets, some placebo-effect can be expected. However, no scientific evidence of any usefulness of this method has been shown.

In conclusion, all the above-described non-diagnostic tests for allergy may result in misleading, even dangerous advice (Fig. 8) (such as malnutrition of the child), and their use is not advised. As a pediatric allergist it is necessary to protect children against all these non-scientific methods. These tests should be frankly criticized, for they are based on dishonest theories and are mainly in use because of huge financial benefits for their prescribers.

Treatment of allergy

The treatment of allergic diseases is largely based on controlling symptoms, which includes the administration of symptomatic medications, such as antihistamines, corticosteroids, beta-agonists, and others. However, once these treatments are withheld, symptoms usually re-occur, as these treatments do not really cure allergy. This is also the case for more specific anti-allergic treatments: once stopped, the symptoms usually re-occur. An exception to this is immunotherapy, which has been shown to have an important long-lasting effect (i.e. carry-over effect), which may persist after stopping the treatment.

In this chapter, a number of more specific approaches to treating allergy will be discussed. These include the role of allergen avoidance, bacterial products, immunotherapy, and anti-IgE.

1. The role of allergen avoidance

When a patient is allergic to a specific allergen, allergen avoidance is the logical recommendation. This approach will not only prevent allergic symptoms from getting worse, but there is also data showing that this can prevent further progression of the Allergic March. However, when discussing allergen avoidance, distinction needs to be made between primary prevention, secondary prevention, and tertiary prevention, because the different phases of prevention need a different approach. In particular, there is a huge difference between primary prevention and secondary-tertiary prevention, as both are totally different and require a totally opposite approach.

Phases of prevention

- **Primary prevention**: refers to the prevention of allergic sensitization in healthy subjects. Usually, it relates to the prevention of the occurrence of allergy (i.e. IgE-production) in healthy newborn babies from allergic families.
- **Secondary prevention** means the prevention of further deterioration (i.e. increase) of allergy in an already sensitized child. Usually, this type of prevention refers to stopping the Allergic March. An example of secondary prevention is the prevention of asthma in a child with eczema or the prevention of asthma in children with allergic rhinitis.

- **Tertiary prevention** means the prevention of symptoms in allergic children with an established allergic disease, such as asthma or rhinitis. It means preventing the worsening of asthma or rhinitis or eczema by preventing the occurrence of underlying allergic reactions.

The role of allergen avoidance in primary prevention

Although it was generally accepted for a long time that early allergen exposure increases the risk of developing allergic diseases, the direct evidence for this statement was weak and certainly not based on controlled, prospective studies, at least not in the case of inhaled allergens. Furthermore, most studies on house dust mite avoidance programs early in life (i.e. avoiding dust contact in newborn babies from allergic families) did **not** show any positive results. Moreover, in recent studies on primary prevention, it was shown that there is no relationship between early exposure to dust (during the first two months of life) and asthma or house dust mite allergy at the age of five and a half years, suggesting that the reduction of dust exposure alone early in life is unlikely to have a major impact of decreasing the incidence of subsequent sensitization to house dust mites.

A number of studies have been published on the effect of outdoor allergens, such as pollen, on early sensitization. In these studies it was demonstrated that early contact to pollen (i.e. children born during the pollen season) increases the risk of developing pollen allergy subsequently in life, suggesting that early contact with an allergen is able to influence the subsequent allergic profile of a subject.

Studies on early exposure to pets give contradictory, sometimes confusing results, although most recent studies have shown that exposure to high levels of cat or dog allergen (Fig. 9) is protective for allergy, and can induce tolerance. The results are more striking for cat than for dog allergen. The timing, dose, duration, and the child's constitution all play a role. For obvious reasons, the prospective controlled study on pet exposure during early life has not been done, and probably will never be done. Similarly, the role of pet exposure during pregnancy has never been properly studied.

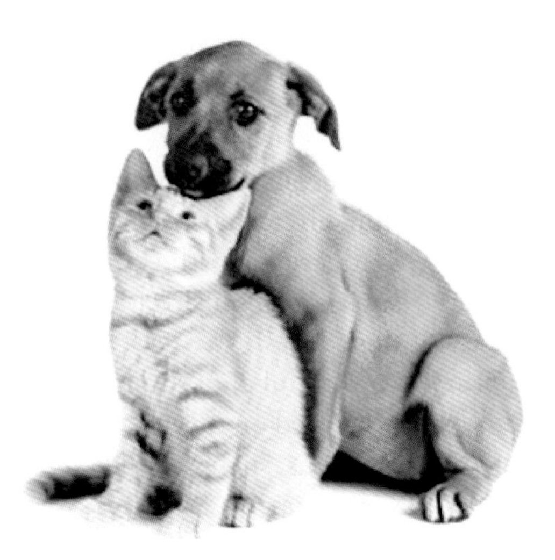

Fig. 9 The first weeks of life with a cat or a dog might result in protection against the subsequent development of allergy in certain children.

In one study by our group, it was found that prenatal exposure to dogs (and not postnatal exposure) was associated with a higher prevalence of eczema in offspring during their second year of life.

It is generally accepted that early introduction of food allergens can lead to an increased allergic sensitization to foods such as cow's milk, egg, and peanuts. Therefore, it is recommended that solid foods be introduced late in life and to exclusively breast feed until six months of age, especially in infants from allergic families. The American Academy of Pediatrics suggests delaying solids until six months of age, cow's milk until one year, egg until two years, and peanuts, tree nuts, and fish until three years. However, only limited scientific data exists on the subject, and these recommendations are certainly not based on extensive prospective studies. In contrast, not all studies could show that early avoidance of foods decreased the risk for the subsequent development of allergic diseases, and the results of a recent study do not support the recommendations given by present feeding guidelines. Moreover, in a recent study from our group on fish allergy, we found a low prevalence of fish allergy in Singaporean children, as compared to the prevalence rates of fish allergy in Europe and the USA. This occurred despite very early introduction of fish in the infant's diet (50% by the 6th month of life) and a high consumption of fish in Singaporean children. These epidemiological data suggest that early introduction of fish and high intake of fish **might protect** against fish allergy, by inducing tolerance and/or anergy to fish instead of allergy.

The role of prenatal allergen exposure, such as from foods and inhalants is very difficult to study, and up till now, very limited information is available. However, from a limited number of studies, it seems that: 1. Prenatal sensitization to allergens, such as house dust mites, pollen, and cow's milk, does occur (through placenta and amniotic fluid), and 2. Allergen avoidance/exposure during pregnancy might influence the Th1-Th2 balance of newborns. For obvious ethical reasons, controlled studies on the role of allergen exposure during pregnancy cannot be performed. Therefore, the impact of prenatal allergen exposure on the allergic sensitization of a child is very difficult to assess, and further understanding of the problem will have to result from indirect data (i.e. animal models or cross-sectional, comparative studies, and not from intervention studies).

Has early allergen exposure changed in recent years?

There is no data showing that early allergen exposure has increased during the last two decades. In contrast, it was since the early eighties that extensive allergen avoidance programs (i.e. food and inhalant allergens) have been instituted all over the world. Despite these programs, allergy to house dust mites and allergic diseases caused by house dust mites have increased. Very often, doctors advise pregnant women from allergic families to institute house dust avoidance measures during pregnancy and during the immediate postnatal period. However, it is now clear that it is impossible to avoid exposure to house dust mites completely, as house dust mites are universally dispersed. Therefore, it could be that the institution of avoidance programs since the early eighties has resulted in exposure to lower, minimal amounts of house dust mites during the first months of life. In animal studies, it has been demonstrated that low allergen exposure preferentially induces IgE-production and not IgG production. Therefore, it is suggested that early and very high exposure to inhaled allergens is associated with protection against allergic sensitization. Many studies now point to the bell-shape relationship – **bell-shape curve** - between exposure and allergic sensitization in newborns: a high exposure and a very low exposure (no exposure) to an inhaled allergen both decrease the risk for allergic sensitization. The problem is that the exact window of sensitization (i.e. timing, concentration) has not been determined, as it is impossible to measure how much of an antigen comes into contact with the immune system of a newborn baby.

Since the early eighties, parents of newborns were often advised to remove their cat or dog. This also may have resulted in an increased risk of developing IgE-mediated hypersensitivity due to exposure to small amounts of dog and cat allergen, and less exposure to bacteria.

In conclusion, **allergen avoidance in primary prevention has not been shown to be effective.** Trying to avoid allergens, such as house dust mites by extensive cleaning of the baby's bedroom (Fig. 10), may result in exposure to small amounts of house dust mites, which may preferentially induce IgE production, leading to an increased risk of allergic sensitization. Furthermore, it seems unlikely that one type of primary prevention (i.e. avoidance of exposure) is suitable for all newborns, as it might be that primary prevention should be tailored to the genes of the child (i.e. genotype). However, at the moment allergic genotype is impossible to determine. It is therefore not recommended to avoid inhaled allergens in all newborns from allergic or non-allergic families.

The role of allergen avoidance in secondary and tertiary prevention

Once IgE-mediated sensitization has occurred, maximum efforts should be undertaken to avoid further contact with the specific antigen, as this will increase the severity of the allergic reactions

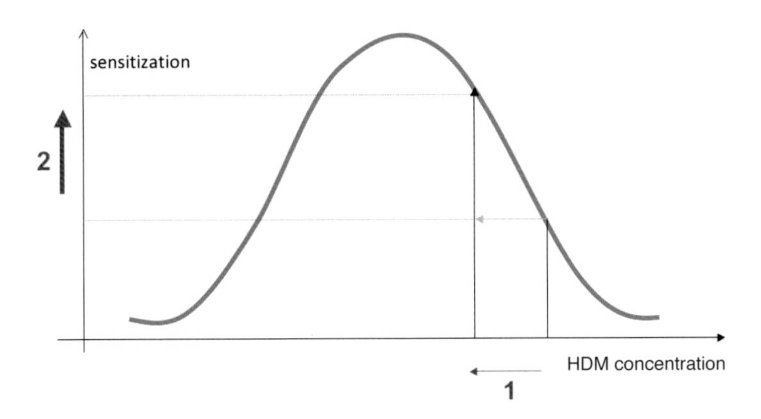

Fig. 10 The effect of allergen removal. Attempts to avoid house dust mites (HDM) (1), such as cleaning the bedroom of a newborn baby, may result in an increased sensitization to house dust mites (2).

and the severity of the allergic symptoms, such as asthma. Directed allergy avoidance can provide considerable benefit to patients. However, complete avoidance is not achievable (even for food allergens), but fortunately, even reducing exposure will decrease the symptoms. This has been shown in a large number of studies on food allergens and inhaled allergens.

1. Allergen avoidance also decreases non-specific airway reactivity.

Several years ago, doctors studied patients with pure grass pollen-induced asthma. These patients wheezed in the spring (April to July), but felt fine in winter. The doctors brought the patients into the laboratory and had them inhale grass pollen (which they were allergic to) and histamine, which is a non-specific trigger of the airways. It was found that it took a lot more histamine to make these patients wheeze in January than it did in June. That is why reducing exposure to allergens also reduced non-specific hypersensitivity of the airways, such as sensitivity to pollution,

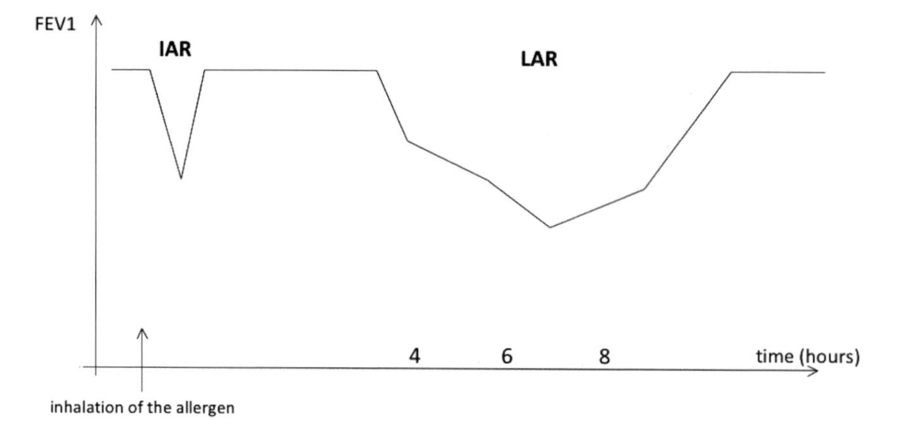

Fig. 11 Inhalation of an allergen can induce 2 consecutive types of bronchial obstructive reactions: an early or immediate asthmatic reaction (IAR), occurring minutes after the inhalation, and a late asthmatic reaction (LAR), occurring 4 – 8 hours after inhalation. The IAR is mainly represents mast cell activation (a bronchoconstriction) , while the LAR represents inflammation (persistent bronchial obstruction).

exercise, and viruses. That is also the reason why reduction of exposure to an allergen will result in less sensitive airways to viral infections (fewer colds, even less wheezing after colds).

2. Allergen exposure can result in late reactions

Many patients get confused because their allergies occur hours after exposure. This is called a "late phase reaction." It was originally described in bakers, who would wake during the night with wheezing. When they were brought into the laboratory and challenged with flour, they again woke up during the night. This *late phase reaction,* starting four to six hours after allergen exposure, is mainly a result of inflammation in the airways (asthma, rhinitis) or skin (eczema), and should be preferentially treated with corticosteroids. It is also the late phase reaction, being the equivalent of inflammation, that is responsible for severe or persistent asthma, as in daily life inhalation of allergens does not occur at one time point, but chronically, especially for the inhalation of house dust mites.

2. The role of bacterial products

The increase of allergic diseases during the last 30 years has been associated with a decrease in bacterial load (i.e. the Hygiene Hypothesis) resulting in less stimulation of the immune system (i.e. less Th1 features). The gastrointestinal system, which comprises the largest lymphoid tissue and in which live most commensal microorganisms, has received more attention during the last few years as a potential stimulator of Th1 immune responses, and as an inhibiting determiner of the development of allergic diseases. How the body maintains homeostasis with an incredibly complex enteric microflora is now beginning to be discerned. Alterations in the intestinal microflora have been detected both in infants suffering from allergic disease and in those later developing the disorder. Delay in the compositional development of lactobacilli and bifidobacteria in gut microflora was a general finding in allergic children.

Therefore, it was postulated that altering/increasing bacterial load early in life might have a suppressing effect on the development of allergy in a young genetically-predisposed child. With this principle in mind, a number of studies have been performed on the administration of bacterial products in children, aiming to prevent (primary prevention) or to inhibit (secondary-tertiary prevention) the development of allergic reactions.

What are the bacterial products that are used to modify allergic diseases?

The bacterial products can be divided into three groups: probiotics (Fig. 12), prebiotics, and synbiotics.

Probiotics are living, "good," or "friendly" bacteria that are similar to those normally found in your body. One widely used definition, developed by the World Health Organization and the Food and Agriculture Organization of the United Nations, is that probiotics are "live microorganisms, which when administered in adequate amounts confer a health benefit on the host". Probiotics are not the same as **prebiotics,**

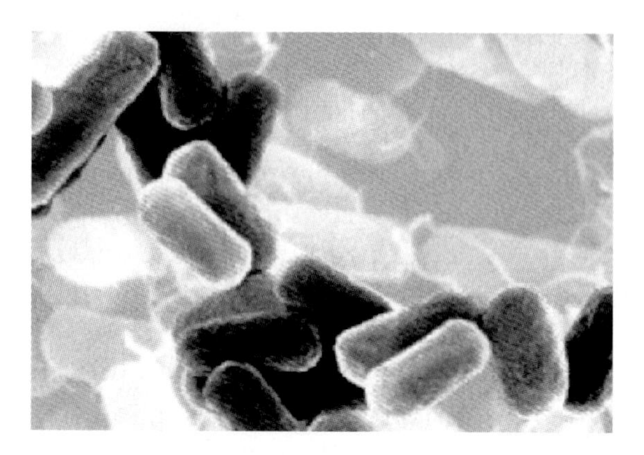

Fig. 12 Probiotics are friendly, living bacteria, similar to those living in our intestine, that are constantly stimulating the immune system into a Th1 direction (i.e. non-allergic direction).

which are non-digestible food ingredients, usually small sugars (oligosaccharides) that selectively stimulate the growth and/or activity of beneficial microorganisms already in people's colons. When probiotics and prebiotics are mixed together, they form **synbiotics**. Probiotics are available in foods and dietary supplements (e.g. capsules, tablets, and powders), and in some other forms as well. Examples of foods containing probiotics are yogurt, fermented and unfermented milk, and some juices and soy beverages. In probiotic foods and supplements, the bacteria may have been present originally or added during preparation. Most probiotics are bacteria similar to those naturally found in people's guts, especially in those of breastfed infants (who have natural protection against many diseases). Most often, the bacteria come from two groups, *Lactobacillus* or *Bifidobacteria*. Within each group, there are different species (e.g. *Lactobacillus acidophilus* and *Bifidobacterium bifidus*), and within each species, different strains (or varieties). A few common probiotics, such as *Saccharomyces boulardii*, are yeasts, which differ from bacteria. Some probiotic foods date back to ancient times, such as fermented foods and cultured milk products. Interest in probiotics in general has been growing. American spending on probiotic supplements, for example, nearly tripled from 1994 to 2003.

Effect of bacterial products on allergic diseases

A number of studies have been performed on the effect of bacterial products on allergic diseases. Unfortunately, contradictory results have been published and the literature on the subject is still confusing. In general, it seems that the effect of bacterial products is more pronounced in primary prevention than in secondary-tertiary prevention. Furthermore, the beneficial effect on eczema is more obvious than on respiratory allergies (asthma, rhinitis).

1. Bacterial products in primary prevention

In the classical study from Finland, published in the Lancet in 2000, by the group of Isolauri, peri-natal administration (during pregnancy and during the first months of life) of lactobacilli halved the subsequent development of eczema during the first two years of life. In most of the children, the administration of probiotics was in association with breast-feeding. However, despite the clinical effect, there was no effect on underlying IgE-mediated hypersensitivity, suggesting that probiotics prevent eczema by other mechanisms than preventing IgE-mediated hypersensitivity. Other studies on the effect of probiotics on primary prevention show contradictory results. Some studies were negative (including a study of our group in Singapore), while other studies from Australia showed an increase in allergic sensitization in newborns who took probiotics. Studies on prebiotics and synbiotics came up with similar results: a significant prevention of eczema in newborns, but less effect on the prevention of respiratory allergies. Taken together, it seems that certain bacterial products are able to prevent the development of eczema, but not of allergic sensitization or respiratory allergy. Bacterial products seem to be more effective when started prenatally (administered to the pregnant woman) and if given in combination with prolonged breast-feeding, and it seems that they merely improve the quality of breast milk.

2. *Bacterial products in secondary-tertiary prevention*

Studies on the effect of bacterial products in the treatment (i.e. secondary-tertiary prevention) of allergic diseases have focused on the early manifestations of allergy, such as food allergy and eczema. Most of the studies were performed with probiotics, showing mild positive effects on eczema and symptoms of food allergy. Studies in older subjects with established asthma or rhinitis have failed to show any improvement. This finding is consistent with findings from animal studies in which bacterial products have more significant effects when immune responses are still developing than once sensitization is established.

Despite several promising findings, the exact role and underlying mechanisms of gut microbiota and/or bacterial products in the development of allergy remain to be elucidated. For successful interventions, more data concerning a communication between host and specific microbial species is needed. However, the inhibiting effect of probiotics on the development of eczema has now been shown in a number of controlled studies. The challenge for the future, however, will be to elucidate the immune mechanisms involved, to determine the best window of exposure, and to determine the dose and type of probiotics that will ensure maximal effectiveness and safety. *In summary*, there is currently still insufficient data on the usage of bacterial products to recommend this as a part of standard therapy in any allergic disease or for the prevention of allergic diseases. Although there has been early promise in atopic dermatitis (eczema), it is generally accepted that more studies are needed to confirm this, and that any benefits are not likely to be great. However, faced with the stress and severe discomfort that can be associated with atopic dermatitis, many families are still choosing to try bacterial products in conjunction with their prescribed treatment. Although the bacterial preparations are generally safe, it is possible that some products could contain milk products and may cause allergic reactions in children with cow's milk allergy. The latter observation provides a cautionary note amid the continuing public enthusiasm for bacterial products.

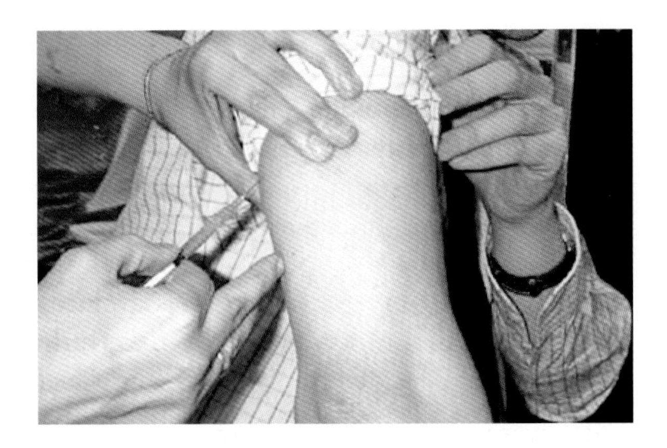

Fig. 13 SIT: In SIT (subcutaneous immunotherapy) the allergen is administered by injection.

3. The role of immunotherapy

Immunotherapy is the only type of treatment that has a carry-over effect, or curative effect, in allergic diseases, as it is the only treatment that is able to permanently suppress underlying allergic reactions. This is in contrast with all other types of medical treatments, which are totally focused on suppressing the symptoms of allergy. Once these latter treatments are stopped, symptoms of allergy will usually re-occur.

The principle of immunotherapy is to desensitize the patient to a particular allergen by administrating increasing doses of the allergen, thereby altering the immune system's response to an offending allergen. Immunotherapy aims to suppress inflammatory reactions that are caused by IgE-mediated hypersensitivity. Currently, two types of immunotherapy are still in use: subcutaneous immunotherapy (SIT) (Fig. 13), which is mainly in use in the USA, and sublingual immunotherapy (SLIT), which is now mainly in use in Europe, but becoming more popular in Asian countries.

1. SIT or subcutaneous immunotherapy

SIT (i.e. subcutaneous injections of allergen) is still widely used in the USA, but less in Europe, where it is now replaced more and more by sublingual immunotherapy (SLIT). SIT is an old treatment, which was introduced more than 100 years ago. The principle is that by administering increasing doses of allergen, the body becomes less allergic and tolerant to the allergen. The underlying mechanisms of SIT (also of SLIT) have not been fully discovered, but it has been shown that a number of immunological changes occur in allergic subjects who receive SIT. These changes include:

a. **a switch from Th2 to Th1 cytokine profile of lymphocytes, resulting in a decrease of allergic reactions**
b. **a suppression of inflammatory cell reactivity, resulting in decreased inflammatory reactions of end organs (lungs, nose, skin)**
c. **production of "good" IgG antibodies, the so-called "blocking antibodies", resulting in tolerance to the allergen**

In a large number of clinical studies performed in adults and children suffering from allergic asthma and allergic rhinitis, it was shown that SIT is effective using standardized extracts of house dust mites and different pollen (but much less effective with cat or dog extracts). Furthermore, in a large review (i.e. Cochrane Review - **The Cochrane Library),** a positive effect of SIT on asthma symptoms and on the usage of anti-asthmatic medication was shown.

Side effects of SIT

Severe side effects have been reported, but do occur rarely, in about two to four percent of patients undergoing SIT. Therefore, caution is still the rule: SIT treatment should be started after careful consideration of every pro and con, and should only be administered by physicians who have sufficient experience with SIT. Some investigators claim that SIT should only be given to patients suffering from severe allergic disease, applying the rule "disease more severe than treatment" (e.g. not in children suffering from mild asthma and/ or mild rhinitis). However, most reported side effects seem to occur in patients in whom SIT is not appropriately administrated and are linked to the lack of experience and competency of medical staff. Reported side effects of SIT are mild allergic reactions (local reaction, rhinitis, and urticaria), asthmatic reactions, and anaphylactic shock. Most side effects occur within 30 minutes after administration and during rush or semi-rush procedures (in some studies up to 35% of patients showed severe local reactions during rush procedures). Therefore, appropriate materials and appropriate protocols for treating every possible side effect should always be available (epinephrine, nebulizer, corticosteroids, etc). The risk of side effects and the fact that SIT is a painful treatment were reasons that in many children SIT has now been replaced by sublingual immunotherapy (SLIT).

Additional effects of SIT

Compared to the pharmaceutical treatment of allergic diseases (i.e. different medications) a number of additional effects of SIT have been demonstrated, pointing to the curative and carry-over effect of SIT. These additional effects contribute substantially to the advantages of SIT as compared to "classical medication treatments".

1. **Prevention of further allergic sensitization**. In a number of studies it was shown that early administration of SIT in young allergic children prevents sensitization to other allergens.
2. **Prevention of asthma in rhinitics**. Studies have demonstrated that SIT prevents the development of asthma and restores bronchial hyperreactivity in children and adults suffering from allergic rhinitis.
3. **Long-term improvement of allergic asthma**. SIT was able to improve the long-term prognosis of allergic asthma in children suffering from house dust mite or grass pollen allergy, increasing the chance to grow out of asthma.

The additional effects of SIT have also been shown in patients receiving SLIT (see below). However, there are more long-term follow-up studies with SIT than with SLIT, and follow-up with SIT is longer than with SLIT (SIT is an older treatment). Despite, less data with SLIT are available, it

1

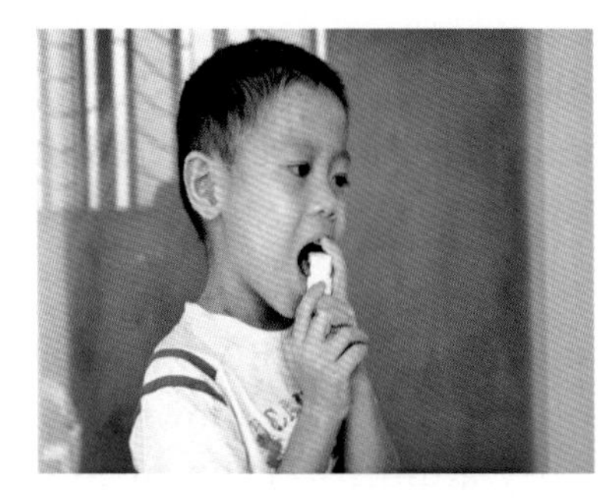

2

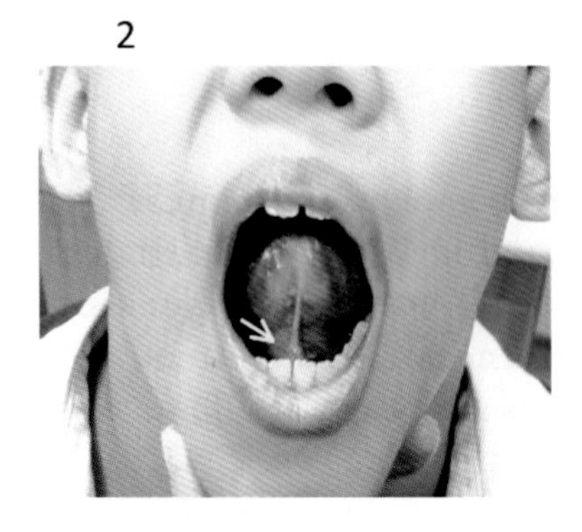

Fig. 14 SLIT in a child. The allergen is put under tongue and kept their for at least 2 minutes, allowing absorption of the allergen through the sublingual mucosa (1) Sometimes a mild sublingual swelling occurs, which is reversible and not dangerous, being the major side effect of SLIT (2).

is suggested that the mechanisms of SIT and SLIT are very similar. Therefore, it is expected that the long-term effects of SLIT are comparable with those of SIT.

2. SLIT or sublingual immunotherapy

SLIT (i.e. sublingual administration of allergen) has a number of advantages compared to SIT, including the following: it is painless, it can be taken at home, and there is far less risk of side effects, especially for severe side effects (some minor side effects can occur, such as mild swelling under the tongue and gastric discomfort). Children apply the drops daily (or three times a week) under their tongue (sublingually) and hold it for two minutes before swallowing (Fig. 14). The mechanisms of SLIT are comparable with those of SIT, and the immunological changes that can be observed in children receiving SLIT are comparable to those in children receiving SIT (i.e. switch from TH2 to Th1, anti-inflammatory effects, and the production of blocking IgG), although the initial immune response involves different cells (dendritic cells in SLIT versus macrophages in SIT). Furthermore, as the sublingual mucosa does not contain any mast cells, the risk for a severe anaphylaxis is very low in SLIT. A large number of clinical studies on SLIT have shown effectiveness in children and adults. From the different studies, the following conclusions can be drawn:

1. SLIT is mainly effective in allergic rhinitis and allergic conjunctivitis. SLIT is less effective in asthma, and has very low effectiveness in eczema.
2. SLIT is effective using extracts of pollen and house dust mites (no studies have shown effectiveness for other allergens, although the first studies on food allergy have produced encouraging results).
3. The optimal duration of SLIT seems to be four years.
4. SLIT has an important carry-over effect of more than five years after stopping SLIT.

SLIT or SIT?

Administering the allergen by mouth (i.e. SLIT), rather than by injection, should decrease the costs of immunotherapy by reducing the need for medical and nursing time, as well as consumables such as syringes, needles, etc. However, it has been calculated that the cumulative dose of allergen for SLIT needs to be 20 to 375 times higher than the usual cumulative doses of allergen given by SIT. The increased cost of allergen extracts is in part offset by reduced consumable and staff costs, but formal cost-benefit analysis is still needed.

The arguments in favor of SLIT are: 1. it works in adults and children, as evidenced by a number of independent trials of single agents, and is child-friendly (no painful injections), 2. it is a safe treatment, 3. it may be cheaper although the reduced costs of administration and reduced need for medical supervision are offset by the increased costs of allergen extracts, and 4. SLIT offers a number of logistical advantages in countries where access to allergy specialists is difficult.

The argument against SLIT is that there are good alternatives, such as that SIT is an old effective treatment having better scientific data than SLIT (more studies on SIT, more long-term data on SIT). However, direct comparison between SIT and SLIT to standard drug therapy is also needed. Only a limited number of studies are available in which SLIT was compared with SIT. Most of the studies are hampered by the lack of a placebo group or by the lack of being blinded. However, in a recent study, using a double-blind, placebo-controlled and double-dummy study design, it was shown that the effectiveness of SLIT was almost similar to the effectiveness of SIT. One of the main conclusions of the study was that the long-term efficacy and preventive capacity as well as the cost-effectiveness of SLIT should be evaluated in large-scale clinical studies before a general introduction as a disease modifying treatment.

4. The role of anti-IgE

In recent years, novel therapeutic strategies have become available for the treatment of allergic diseases. These treatments include neutralizing products for mediators and cytokines, free immunoglobulin light chains, and anti-IgE (omaluzimab). Most of these treatments are still in an experimental phase (under study) and not yet suitable for daily use in the treatment of allergic diseases in children. However, in the near future it might be that these products will become available in the management of allergic diseases.

Omalizumab (anti-IgE) is a recombinant humanized monoclonal antibody targeted against IgE, blocking the effect of IgE. Omalizumab causes a reduction in total serum IgE in allergic patients, which attenuates the amount of antigen-specific IgE that can bind to and sensitize tissue mast cells and basophiles. This, in turn, leads to a decrease in the symptoms of allergic diseases. The monoclonal antibody contains 5% murine sequences (needed for the IgE binding portion) and 95% human residues from a human IgG molecule. Omalizumab reduces the amount of free IgE (the unbound form present in the circulation) available to bind to receptors and results in a reduction in the expression of high affinity IgE receptors. Omalizumab does not bind to IgE already bound to effector cells.

Usually, omalizumab is administrated subcutaneously, at monthly intervals. In clinical trails, omalizumab reduces asthma exacerbations and symptoms in patients suffering from allergic asthma and has a low anaphylactic potential. When added to existing therapy, patients treated with omalizumab had a quarter the rate of clinically significant asthma exacerbations. The GINA (Global Initiative for Asthma) has recognized the role of anti-IgE therapy in treating adults and older children (> 12 years) with severe persistent asthma. Initiation of anti-IgE therapy is now recommended for these patients at step four of GINA guidelines, i.e. in severe asthma. Severe asthma has a major impact on health-care resource utilization. To date, treatment options have been limited in this target population. Omalizumab reduces symptoms, exacerbations, and emergency visits in patients who are not adequately controlled on inhaled corticosteroids and long-acting beta agonists. It is a valuable therapeutic option, addressing an unmet need in the area of severe asthma. A major disadvantage of omalizumab is its high cost and the fact that it is only a controller treatment: once stopped the symptoms may re-occur. Omalizumab has yet not been studied in younger children or in children suffering from severe eczema or rhino-sinusitis.

In clinical practice, the use of omalizumab should be limited to those patients, aged 12 to 75 years, with moderate to severe persistent allergic asthma, who: 1) are inadequately controlled with appropriate combination therapy; 2) have complications due to inhaled or oral corticosteroid use; 3) have increased need for urgent care, emergency department or inpatient services due to asthma exacerbations; 4) have significant impairment in activities of daily living; or 5) have unresolved adherence issues. Omalizumab should be administered every two to four weeks by subcutaneous injection based on body weight and total serum IgE levels. Omalizumab should not be used off-label until appropriate dosages and adverse event potential are adequately assessed.

12

General Conclusion - The Future of Allergic Diseases in Children

In recent years, allergic diseases have become a major problem in children, affecting more than 20% to 30% of them worldwide. The increase of allergic diseases was most pronounced during the 1980s and 1990s. From the start of the 21st century, a plateau phase in prevalence of allergic diseases has occurred in most countries, exhibiting even a slight decrease (mainly of asthma) in a number of countries. However, taken together, allergic diseases are responsible for a considerable level of morbidity, leading to a high financial burden. Most allergic diseases can be controlled, although in some children allergy has a large impact on their quality of life, and in a minority, allergy can be fatal.

Current knowledge on allergic diseases has improved considerably. However, there are still a lot of issues that need to be explored and for which we need more and better scientific evidence. Still, too often, allergic diseases in children are the subject of a non-scientific approach (diagnosis and treatment), leading to misconception, confusion and over-expectation in parents, as it is only by **a correct scientific approach** (i.e. scientific studies) that we will be able to really help children. In this chapter the future of allergic diseases will be discussed briefly. In a second part, current knowledge on primary prevention will be overviewed.

The future approaches and future treatments

There are still many issues on allergic diseases in children that need to be explored, as current knowledge is still very limited. It is not the scope of this text to go into the details, and to describe all the different studies that still need to be performed. However, certain main topics can be identified. The topics can be divided into diagnostic topics (also covering mechanisms and pathophysiology) and therapeutic topics (focusing on the control and cure of allergic diseases). Briefly, the following are the main fields that need to be studied in the near future:

a) On the diagnosis of allergic diseases:

1. We need to learn more about the genetics and the impact of the environment on gene expression, especially the role of the environment during pregnancy and in early life. This will enable us to identify the risk factors more adequately, and to start treatment (or prevention) early in life.

2. We need to know more about the many faces of allergic expression. Why is it that some children are very allergic and have no symptoms? Why is it that other children with only a mild allergy will develop severe asthma or severe eczema? Why it is that children of the same parents can show different types of allergy?
3. We need to know more about the natural evolution of allergic diseases in children. What makes an allergic disease persist and why is it that a large number of children grow out of their allergic diseases? What makes a child grow out of an allergic disease (i.e. the mechanisms of growing out of a disease)?

b) On the treatment of allergic diseases:

1. We should develop better controller treatments with high efficacy and no side effects. Furthermore, all controller treatments should be child friendly, easy to administer, cheap, and accessible to every child worldwide.
2. We should develop treatments that can cure children with allergy, such as immunotherapy (e.g. SLIT). These treatments should have a long-lasting effect, without side effects on the immune system of the child. Furthermore, these treatments should fulfill the same conditions as any controller treatment (see above).

Prevention of allergic diseases: "what can I do to prevent my newborn baby from becoming allergic?"

Preventing allergy from occurring or preventing allergic sensitization in a healthy newborn is called **primary prevention**. Often, allergic parents consult a doctor, asking him to prevent allergy from occurring in their healthy newborn, and often the doctor will have to admit that this is a very difficult task, mainly because allergy is a genetic disease and not much can be done by trying to manipulate the environment. However, recently a number of important observations have been made, showing that allergic manifestations can at least be partially prevented or postponed.

Until recently, primary prevention was mainly based on the assumption that allergen avoidance (foods and inhalants) is the most effective measure to prevent allergic sensitization and its consequences. Based on this, studies on primary prevention measures have specifically targeted nutrition and environmental control in newborn babies (Table 1).

Table 1 Primary Prevention Strategies and their Outcome

Strategy	Outcome (long-term)
Prolonged breast feeding	Breast feeding is useful for the child's health and may prevent allergic sensitization in early life. However, there is no clear benefit for preventing the development of inhalant allergies later in childhood.
Hydrolyzed formula feeding (HA-milks)	Hydrolyzed formulas in young at-risk infants reduces the incidence of food allergy and eczema up to the ages of three to five years, but has no benefit beyond the sixth month of life.
Delayed introduction of solid foods	There is no evidence that the delayed introduction of solid food after six to eight months of life is useful for preventing food allergy.
Avoidance of indoor inhaled allergens	Contradictory results. Reduction of exposure to indoor allergens in newborn babies (house dust mites) might even increase the risk for allergy and asthma.
Avoidance of pollution and smoke	Pollution and smoke avoidance is mandatory to maintain respiratory health, and may be effective in reducing the risk of asthma and allergy.

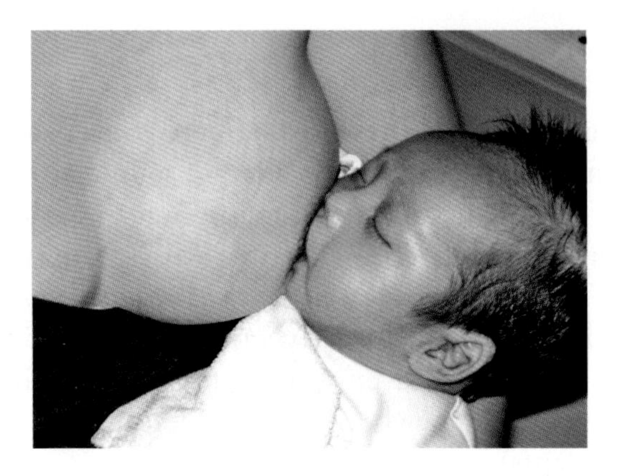

Fig. 1 A breast-fed baby. Breast feeding is still the best way to prevent the development of allergy.

The most striking results on primary prevention have been shown for prolonged breast feeding (Fig. 1) and for the avoidance of pollution and smoke.

Apart of this, other measures, such as hydrolyzed formulas or late introduction of solid foods showed far less convincing results. Furthermore, avoidance of inhalant allergen exposure showed contradictory results, even leading to increased sensitization to these allergens.

The role of bacterial products in primary prevention is now intensively studied. Most studies on probiotics, prebiotics and synbiotics show positive results. However, some of the studies were negative and in other studies an increase of allergic sensitization was demonstrated. Therefore, more studies are needed on bacterial products before general recommendations can be given.

In conclusion, many more studies are needed on primary prevention and on the early events of allergic diseases, addressing the following issues:

1. The mechanisms of the initiation of allergic reactions in newborns (i.e. which molecules are responsible for the start of allergy)
2. The exact profiles of the genes that are involved in allergic

reactions to different allergens (foods, inhalant allergens)

3. The exact role of bacterial products (probiotics, prebiotics, and synbiotics), including the best type of bacterial product, best dose, and best window of administration
4. The exact role of early allergen exposure, including whether high allergen exposure is able to induce tolerance to allergens (including the role of early administration of immunotherapy, including SLIT)

Allergic Diseases in the Future: Aims for Approach

- All allergic children worldwide should receive optimal and early treatment for allergy, enabling them to have a healthy life.
- Because of the high prevalence of allergy, every newborn baby should be screened for allergy. According to the risk, optimal primary prevention should be able to decrease the development of subsequent allergic disease.

Common Questions Asked by Parents on Allergy

1) **If a family member is prone to allergies and develop an allergic illness (asthma, sinus etc), would the chances of their children having an allergy be higher?**

   Yes, if the family history is positive for allergy, then the risk for the children to develop allergy is higher. If both parents are highly allergic, almost 100% of their children will develop allergy. If neither of the parents is allergic, the risk is about 15% – 20%. This is because allergy is a complex genetic disease in which a large number of genes are involved. Moreover, children who have allergic rhinitis or asthma (and who are undertreated) become more sensitive to all kinds of viral respiratory infections. This means that they fall sick more often with colds and flu (including fever). These infections settle once a proper treatment is instituted.

2) What should an expecting mother take note of in order to reduce the likelihood of her child falling prey to such illnesses?

Since allergy is a genetic disease, there is little that can be done. Furthermore, recent studies have shown that an unborn child (the fetus) is highly protected during pregnancy, and that the development of allergic reactions in the fetus is suppressed. So, during pregnancy there is little that a mother can do, except to "stay healthy" (eat healthily, and refrain from smoking and from the use of alcohol). See also the chapter on "Primary Prevention of Allergy."

3) For families that have children with such illnesses, at what age do the symptoms usually surface? And what are these symptoms?

Allergy to foods can occur very early in life, even during the first weeks of life. Foods involved in early food allergy are cow's milk, hen's egg, soy and wheat. Other food allergies (peanuts, seafood) usually occurs later in life (during the first 5 years), although a new allergy can start at any age, including adulthood.

Inhalant allergy (house dust mites, pollen, and pets) usually starts later in life, and in most children beyond the age of 2 years. If a child is genetically very allergic, a house dust mite allergy usually starts around the age of 2 years.

4) When a child develops these symptoms, do they appear at the same time or in a progressive manner?

No, symptoms of allergy develop in a specific sequence, although there are exceptions. A typical pattern is "The Allergic March" (see also "The Allergic March" in Chapter 1). In most children, allergy manifests as eczema or gastrointestinal symptoms (vomiting, diarrhea) during the first months of life, followed by asthma (first

5 years of life), and then followed by allergic rhinitis (beyond the age of 4 – 5 years).

5) When our children develop these illnesses, such as rhino-sinusitis, or asthma, what measures can we take?

   A) Take normal prescribed medication and wait for the illness to subside? or

   B) Insist on a stronger dosage of medication for faster cure.

   There is no cure for allergy in most children, and except for immunotherapy (see chapter on "Immunotherapy"), all treatments are controller treatments: this means that the symptoms will re-occur once the treatment is stopped. However, it is important to treat all symptoms as soon as possible, because untreated allergy can induce complications (infections) and has an important negative impact on the quality of life of the child. Treating all symptoms will prevent complications from occurring and will increase the chance of the child growing out of the symptoms. Untreated allergy will lead to more severe allergic diseases and to complications, such as sinusitis, pneumonia, skin infections (with permanent scarring of the skin). My advice to parents: do not accept any symptoms occurring in your child.

6) Many children and infants have taken allergy tests. We would, therefore, like to know the proportion of children developing allergies due to dust mites as compared to those who are allergic due to other causes?

   In the chapter on "Epidemiology," you can find all the data on the prevalence of different allergies in children. In short, house dust mite allergy is the most common allergy in children (especially in Asia), affecting more than 20% to 30% of them. This is especially in children with asthma or rhinitis who have a very high prevalence of house dust mite allergy. In reviewing older children with asthma and rhinitis (beyond the age of 5 years), it can be concluded that almost all of them have a house dust mite allergy.

7) **For those children with allergies to dust mites, what precautions can we take and how effective are these measures?**

Once a child is allergic to house dust mites, it is very important to try to reduce their exposure to house dust mites as much as possible. However, complete avoidance seems impossible. The highest concentrations of house dust mites are found in the bedroom, especially in mattresses and pillows. Therefore, sleeping on old mattresses and pillows should be avoided. Furthermore, extensive cleaning of mattresses and pillows (using a good-quality vacuum cleaner) and washing of sheets and covers is necessary. Sunning the mattress is also recommended. More details on how to avoid house dust mites are given in the chapter on "Allergens" (see house dust mite avoidance).

8) **Why do some people have allergy to certain foods while others are free from food allergy?**

Developing a food allergy is a complicated process, and is dependent on the genetic constitution of a person as well as exposure to the food (age, dose, number of exposures, prenatal exposure (before birth) and postnatal exposure (after birth, early in life)). However, we still don't understand the exact mechanisms and we still can't answer the question why a certain child develops a certain food allergy. Furthermore, the mechanisms are not the same for every food. In general, it is believed that early exposure in life of small amounts could trigger subsequent food allergy. This includes contact with the food through smelling or touching. Exposure to large amounts early in life is more likely to induce tolerance. The risk of developing a food allergy is dependent on the genetic constitution and, therefore, prevention of food allergy is not the same for every child, but should be tailored according to the genetic constitution. Unfortunately, genotyping (i.e. knowing the exact genetic constitution) of food allergy is still largely impossible as we don't know yet the different genes that are involved.

9) How could food allergy be treated? Is there a cure?

Unfortunately, apart from strict avoidance of the food, there is no cure for food allergy. We can treat the symptoms but can't treat or prevent the underlying mechanisms. However, studies are now ongoing focusing on specific types of immunotherapy for food allergy, aiming to desensitize the child. Most studies are now on peanut allergy, but in the future other foods will be studied.

10) How should a parent with a food allergic child manage this child?

Avoidance of the food is the only treatment. This would mean that everybody in contact with the child should know about his or her food allergy (school, babysitter, grandparents, etc). It is also important to be aware of the contents of processed food (read the labels) and to have a complete list of forbidden food products.

References

1. TEXTBOOKS

1. Lockey RF, Bukantz SC. (eds). (1999) *Allergens and Allergen immunotherapy*, 2nd edition, revised and expanded. Marcel Dekker Inc.
2. Silverman M (ed). (2002) *Childhood Asthma and Other Wheezing Disorders*. London, Arnold.
3. Warner J, Jackson WF (eds). (1994) *Color Atlas of Pediatric Allergy.* Mosby-Year Book Europe Limited.
4. Adkinson NF, Yunginger JW, Busse WW, *et al*. (eds). (2003) *Middleton's Allergy. Principles and Practice,* 6th edition. Mosby, Inc.
5. Delves P, Martin S, Burton D, Roitt I. (2006) *Roitt's Essential Immunology*, 11th edition. Blackwell Publishing.
6. Holgate ST, MK. (1993) *Allergy*, 1st edition. C.V. Mosby.
7. Cantani A. (2008) *Pediatric Allergy, Asthma, and Immunology*. Berlin, Springer.

2. INTERNET SITES

There is a lot of information on allergy in children on the Internet (see at Google). Some sites are very good, giving high level scientific information. However, **a considerable number of sites are not good**: they have commercial purposes, give wrong information or focus on new "miracle" treatments. We should all be aware of this! The following sites are recommended for further reading. Most of them are official sites from international or national medical organizations:

- World Allergy Organization (WAO): http://www.worldallergy.org/index.php
- American Academy for Asthma Allergy and Immunology (AAAAI): http://www.aaaai.org/
- European Academy for Allergy and Clinical Immunology (EAACI): http://eaaci.net/site/homepage.php
- Asia Pacific Association of Allergy, Asthma and Clinical Immunology (APAAACI): http://www.apaaaci.org/
- APAPARI (Asian Pediatric Association for Pediatric Allergy, Respirology, and Immunology): http://www.apapari.org/
- UCB-School of Allergy: http://www.theucbinstituteofallergy.com/
- Children's Allergy Network "I CAN!" (Singapore) www.ican.com.sg
- International organization on food allergy: http://www.foodallergy.org/
- Food allergy network (Singapore) http://www.foodallergysingapore.org/Home_Page.html
- PUBMED: is an important site on which all medical literature can be found, using key words. Just type in a key word and you will find a lot of good information on allergic diseases in children. http://www.ncbi.nlm.nih.gov/sites/entrez

3. ARTICLES IN MEDICAL JOURNALS - 10 key references per chapter

I do realize that there is a lot of literature available on the Internet. For this part on references, I have chosen 10 references for each chapter of which I think they are innovative and cover key issues. It was a choice, in which I have tried to be objective. However, I am aware that there are plenty of other articles that I could have been listed here as well.

CHAPTER 1: On allergy and allergic reactions

1. Akdis CA. (2007) An article on recent findings in the pathogenesis of allergy and the immune system: New insights into mechanisms of immunoregulation in 2007. *J Allergy Clin Immunol* **122**: 700–709.
2. Lambrecht BN. (2008) On the role of specific macrophages (dendritic cells) in allergy: Lung dendritic cells: targets for therapy in allergic disease. *Curr Mol Med* **8**: 393–400.
3. Suarez CJ, Parker NJ, Finn PW. (2008) On the role of innate immunity in allergy: Innate immune mechanism in allergic asthma. *Curr Allergy Asthma Rep* **8**: 451–458.
4. Rivera J, Fierro NA, Olivera A, Suzuki R. (2008) *On the role of mast cells:* New insights on mast cell activation via high affinity receptor for IgE. *Adv Immunol* **98**: 85–120.
5. Galli SJ, Tsai M, Piliponsky AM. (2008) *On allergy and inflammation*: The development of allergic inflammation. *Nature* **454**: 445–454.
6. Larché M, Robinson DS, Kay AB. (2003) *On the role of T lymphocytes in asthma and allergy:* The role of T lymphocytes in the pathogenesis of asthma. *J Allergy Clin Immunol* **111**: 450–463.
7. Galli SJ, Tsai M, Piliponsky AM. (2008) On mechanisms of allergy-induced inflammation: The development of allergic inflammation. *Nature* **24**: 445–454.
8. Renz H, Blümer N, Virna S, *et al.* (2006) On Th1 –Th2 balance in allergy: The immunological basis of the hygiene hypothesis. *Chem Immunol Allergy* **91**: 30–48.
9. Elkord E. (2008) On regulatory T cells in allergy: Novel therapeutic strategies by regulatory T cells in allergy. *Chem Immunol Allergy* **94**: 150–157.
10. Steinman L. (2007) A recent overview of the role of Th17-cells: A brief history of Th17, the first major revision in the Th1/Th2 hypothesis of T cell-mediated tissue damage. *Nature Med* **13**: 139–145.

CHAPTER 2: Epidemiology of allergic diseases in Asia

1. Wong GWK, Chow CM. (2008) On the importance of epidemiology and risk factors for asthma: Childhood asthma epidemiology: insights from comparative studies of rural and urban populations. *Pediatr Pulmonol* **43**: 107–116.

2. Eder W, Ege MJ, von Mutius E. (2006) On the epidemiology of asthma: The asthma epidemic. *N Engl J Med* **355**: 2226–2235.
3. Asher MI, Montefort S, Björksten B, *et al.* and the ISAAC Phase Three Study Group. (2006) On epidemiology of asthma, allergic rhinoconjunctivitis, and eczema: Worldwide time trends in the prevalence of symptoms of asthma, allergic rhinoconjunctivitis, and eczema in childhood: ISAAC Phases One and Three repeat multicountry cross-sectional surveys. *Lancet* **368**: 733–743.
4. Wong GWK, Ko FWS, Hui DSC, *et al.* (2004) An article on epidemiology of asthma in three Chinese cities: Factors associated with difference in prevalence of asthma in children from three cities in China: multicentre epidemiological survey. *Br Med J* **329**: 486–489.
5. Sears MR, Greene JM, Willan AR, *et al.* (2003) A long-term study on the evolution of asthma: A longitudinal, population-based, cohort study of childhood asthma followed to adulthood. *N EnglJ Med* **349**: 1414–1422.
6. Lee BW, Shek L P-C, Gerez IFA, *et al.* (2008) On food allergy in Asia: Food Allergy – Lessons from Asia. *World Allergy:* 129–133.
7. Tan TN, Lim DL-C, Lee BW, Van Bever HP. (2005) On epidemiology of allergic diseases in young children in Singapore: Prevalence of allergy-related symptoms in the second year of life. *Ped Allergy Immunol* **16**: 151–6.
8. Stensen L, Thomsen SF, Backer V. (2008) On the epidemiology of eczema: Change in prevalence of atopic dermatitis between 1986 and 2001 among children. *Allergy Asthma Proc* **29**: 392–396.
9. Lin RY, Anderson AS, Shah SN, Nurruzzaman F. (2008) On the epidemiology of anaphylaxis: Increasing anaphylaxis hospitalizations in the first 2 decades of life: New York State, 1990 -2006. *Ann Allergy Asthma Immunol* **101**: 387–393.
10. Demoly P. (2008) On the epidemiology of drug allergy: Drug allergies – unknown dangers to patients. *Expert Opin Drug Saf* 7: 347–350.

CHAPTER 3: The allergens

1. Chapman MD, Ferreira F, Villalba M, *et al.* and the CREATE consortium. (2008) A recent review on standardization of allergens for diagnostic tests and for immunotherapy: The European Union CREATE

Project: A model for international standardization of allergy diagnostics and vaccines. *J Allergy Clin Immunol* **122**: 882–889.
2. Pomés A. (2008) On the structure and biological function of allergens: Allergen structures and biologic functions: the cutting edge of allergy research. *Curr Allergy Asthma Rep* **8**: 425–432.
3. Mari A. (2008) On allergens and on what makes a protein to become an allergen: When does a protein become an allergen? Searching for a dynamic definition based on most advanced technology tools. *Clin Exp Allergy* **38**: 1089–1094.
4. Custovic A, Chapman M. (1998) On house dust mite allergens: Risk levels for mite allergens. Are they meaningful? *Allergy* **53**: 71–76
5. Chua KY, Cheong N, Kuo IC, *et al.* (2007) On the tropical house dust mite, Blomia tropicalis: The Blomia tropicalis allergens. *Protein Pept Lett* **14**: 325–333.
6. Simpson A, Custovic A. (2005) *On pet allergens*: Pets and the development of allergic sensitization. *Curr Allergy Asthma Rep* **5**: 212–220.
7. D'Amato G, Cecchi L, Bonini S, *et al.* (2007) On pollen allergens in Europe: Allergenic pollen and pollen allergy in Europe. *Allergy* **62**: 976–990.
8. Breiteneder H, Mills EN. (2005) Molecular properties of food allergens. *J Allergy Clin Immunol* **115**: 14–23.
9. Zuidmeer L, Goldhahn K, Rona RJ, *et al.* (2008) A review of studies on plant food allergens: The prevalence of plant food allergies: a systematic review. *J Allergy Clin Immunol* **121**: 1210–1218.
10. Fernandez-Rivas M, Gonzalez-Mancebo E, Alonso Diaz de Durana MD. (2008) On allergens in fruits and vegetables: Allergies to fruits and vegetables. *Ped Allergy Immunol* **19**: 675–681.

CHAPTER 4: Asthma in children

1. Van Bever HP, Desager KN, Hagendorens M. (2002) On types, triggers and long-term outcome of childhood asthma: Critical evaluation of prognostic factors in childhood asthma. *Pediatr Allergy Immunol* **12**: 1–9.
2. Castro-Rodriguez JA, Holberg CJ, Wright AL, Martinez FD. (2000) On outcome of different types of asthma in young children: A clinical index to define risk of asthma in young children with recurrent wheezing. *Am J Respir Crit Care Med* **162**: 1403–1406.

3. Martinez FD, Wright AL, Taussig LM, *et al.* and the Group Health Medical Associates. (1995) On asthma in young children: Asthma and wheezing in the first six years of life. *N Engl J Med* 332: 133–138.
4. Martinez FD, Helms PJ. (1998) On the different types of asthma: Types of asthma and wheezing. *Eur Respir J* **12 (Suppl. 27):** 3s–8s.
5. Brand PLP, Baraldi E, Bisgaard H, *et al.* (2008) A review on the different types of asthma in preschool children: Definition, assessment and treatment of wheezing disorders in preschool children: an evidence-based approach. *Eur Respir J* **32**: 1096–1110.
6. Nickel R, Kulig M, Forster J, *et al.* (1997) On the role of allergy in asthma: Sensitization to hen's egg at the age of twelve months is predictive for allergic sensitization to common indoor and outdoor allergens at the age of three years. *J Allergy Clin Immunol* **99**: 613–617.
7. Papadopoulos NG, Kalobatsou A. (2007) On the role of viruses in asthma: Respiratory viruses in childhood asthma. *Curr Opin Allergy Clin Immunol* 7: 91–95.
8. Bacharier LB, Boner A, Carlsen HH, *et al.* (2008) A recent review on the treatment of asthma: Diagnosis and treatment of asthma in childhood: a PRACTALL consensus report. *Allergy* **63**: 5–34.
9. O'Callaghan C, Barry PW. (2000) On different devices for treating asthma: How to choose delivery devices for asthma. *Arch Dis Childh* **82**: 185–187.
10. Roorda RJ, Gerritsen J, van Aalderen WMC, *et al.* (1994) On the long-term prognosis of asthma: Follow-up of asthma from childhood to adulthood: influence of potential childhood risk factors on the outcome of pulmonary function and bronchial responsiveness in adulthood. *J Allergy Clin Immunol* **93**: 575–584.

CHAPTER 5: Allergy of the upper airways and eyes

1. de Groot H, Brand PLP, Fokkens WF, Berger MY. (2007) A review article on rhinoconjunctivitis in children: Allergic rhinoconjunctivitis in children. *Br Med J* **335**: 985–988.
2. Rolinck-Werninghaus C, Keil T, Kopp M, *et al.* and the Omalizumab Rhinitis Study Group. (2008) On seasonal rhinitis and allergy in children: Specific IgE serum concentration is associated with symptom severity in children with seasonal allergic rhinitis. *Allergy* **63**: 1339–1344.

3. Wang DY. (2005) On risk factors for the development of allergic rhinitis: Risk factors of allergic rhinitis: genetic or environmental? *Ther Clin Risk Manag* **1**: 115–123.
4. Muliol J, Maurer M, Bousquet J. (2008) On the impact of allergic rhinitis on sleep: Sleep and allergic rhinitis. *J Investig Allergol Clin Immunol* **18**: 415–419.
5. Chng SY. (2008) An article from Singapore on sleep disorders and rhinitis in children: Sleep disorders in children — the Singapore perspective. *Ann Acad Med Singapore* **37**: 706–709.
6. Baena-Cagnani CE, Passalacqua G, Gómez M, *et al.* (2007) On new treatments for allergic rhinitis: New perspectives in the treatment of allergic rhinitis and asthma in children. *Curr Opin Allergy Clin Immunol* **7**: 201–206.
7. Origlieri C, Bielory L. (2008) On the usage of intranasal corticosteroids in allergic rhinitis: Intranasal corticosteroids and allergic rhinoconjunctivitis. *Curr Opin Allergy Clin Immunol* **8**: 450–456.
8. Simons FE. (2004) On the usage of antihistamines in allergic rhinitis: Advances in H1-antihistamines. *N Engl J Med* **18**: 2203–2217.
9. Abelson MB, Granet D. (2006) On allergic eye diseases (including conjunctivitis) in children: Ocular allergy in pediatric practice. *Curr Allergy Asthma Rep* **6**: 306–311.
10. Novembre E, Mori F, Pucci N, *et al.* (2007) On chronic sinusitis in children: Systemic treatment of rhinosinusitis in children. *Ped Allergy Immunol* **18 (suppl. 18):** 56–61.

CHAPTER 6: Eczema or atopic dermatitis

1. Rancé F, Boguniewicz M, Lau S. (2008) On what is new in eczema (mid-2008): New visions for atopic eczema — an iPAC summary and future trends. *Ped Allergy Immunol* **19 (suppl. 19):** 17–25.
2. Akdis CA, Akdis M, Bieber T, *et al.* (2006) An extensive and good overview article on eczema: Diagnosis and treatment of atopic dermatitis in children and adults — European Academy of Allergology and Clinical Immunology/American Academy of Allergy, Asthma and Immunology / PRACTALL Consensus Report. *J Allergy Clin Immunol* **118**: 152–169.

3. Hanifin JM, Raijka G. (1980) On classification of eczema: Diagnostic features of atopic dermatitis. *Acta Dermatol Venereol (Stockh)* **92**: 44–47.
4. Elias PM, Hatano Y, Williams ML. (2008) On skin barrier abnormalities in eczema: Basis for the barrier abnormality in atopic dermatitis: Outside-inside-outside pathogenic mechanisms. *J Allergy Clin Immunol* **121**: 1337–1343.
5. Cork MJ, Robinson DA, Vasilopoulos Y, *et al.* (2006) An overview of skin barrier abnormalities in eczema: New perspectives on epidermal barrier dysfunction in atopic dermatitis: Gene-environmental interactions. *J Allergy Clin Immunol* **118**: *3–21.*
6. Leung DYM. (2006) On genetics of eczema and on the role of the environment: New insights into the complex gene-environment interactions evolving into atopic dermatitis. *J Allergy Clin Immunol* **118**: 37–39.
7. Flohr C, Johansson SGO, Wahlgren C-F. (2004) On the role of allergy in eczema: How atopic is atopic dermatitis? *J Allergy Clin Immunol* **114**: 150–158.
8. CA, Adkis M, Bieber T, *et al.* (2006) On new treatments of eczema: Akdis; European Academy of Allergology; Clinical Immunology / American Academy of Allergy, Asthma and immunology/ PRACTALL Consensus Report. *Allergy* **61**: 969–987.
9. Krakowski AC, Eichenfield LF, Dohil MA. (2008) On treatment of eczema: Management of atopic dermatitis in the pediatric population. *Pediatrics* **122**: 812–824.
10. Belloni B, Andres C, Ollert M, *et al.* (2008) On new treatments for eczema: Novel immunological approaches in the treatment of atopic eczema. *Curr Opin Allergy Immunol* **8**: 423–427.

CHAPTER 7: Urticaria and angioedema

1. Krishnamurthy A, Naguwa SM, Gershwin ME. (2008) An excellent review on the mechanisms of angioedema in children: Pediatric angioedema. *Clin Rev Allergy Immunol* **34**: 250–259.
2. Deacock SJ. (2008) On the diagnosis and treatment of urticaria in children: An approach to the patient with urticaria. *Clin Exp Immunol* **153**: 151–161.

3. Krishnamurthy A, Naguwa SM, Gershwin ME. (2008) On angioedema in children: Pediatric angioedema. *Clin Rev Allergy Immunol* **34**: 250–259.
4. Greaves MW. (1995) An excellent review on chronic urticaria: Chronic urticaria. *N Engl J Med* **332**: 1767–1772.
5. Novembre E, Cianferoni A, Mori F, *et al.* (2008) A recent review on urticaria in children: Urticaria and urticaria related skin condition/disease in children. *Eur Ann Allergy Clin Immunol* **40**: 5–13.
6. Schad CA, Skoner DP. (2008) On the usage of antihistamines in childhood urticaria: Antihistamines in the pediatric population — achieving optimal outcomes when treating seasonal allergic rhinitis and chronic urticaria. *Allergy Asthma Proc* **29**: *7–13.*
7. Farkas H, Varga L, Széplaki G, *et al.* (2007) On the management of angioedema: Management of hereditary angioedema in pediatric patients. *Pediatrics* **120**: e713–722.
8. Kimata H. (2004) An interesting article on latex allergy in young children: Latex allergy in infants younger than 1 year. *Clin Exp Allergy* **34**: 1910–1915.
9. Martorell A, Sanz J, Ortiz M, *et al.* (2000) A study on dermographism in children: Prevalence of dermographism in children. *J Invest Allergol Clin Immunol* **10**: 166–169.
10. Bailey E, Shaker M. (2008) A recent review article on the treatment of urticaria: An update on childhood urticaria and angioedema. *Curr Opin Pediatr* **20**: 425–430.

CHAPTER 8: Food allergy

1. Lee BW, Shek LP-C, Gerez IFA, *et al.* (2008) On food allergy in Asia: Food Allergy – Lessons from Asia. *World Allergy Journal* **July**: 129–133.
2. Lack G. (2008) An interesting overview on egg allergy: Food Allergy. *New Engl J Med* **359**: 1252–1260.
3. Sampson HA. (1999) A review on the mechanisms and symptoms of food allergy: Food allergy: 1. Immunopathogenesis and clinical disorders. *J Allergy Clin Immunol* **103**: 717–728.

4. Hattevig G, Kjellman B, Björksten B. (1987) On food allergy in young children: Clinical symptoms and IgE responses to common food proteins and inhalants in the first 7 years of life. *Clin Allergy* **17**: 571–578.
5. Sampson HA, Mendelson L, Rosen JP. (1992) On severe reactions to food: Fatal and near-fatal anaphylactic reactions to food in children and adolescents. *N Engl J Med* **327**: 380–384.
6. Kulig M, Bergmann R, Klettke U, *et al.* (1999) On the association between food allergy and allergy to inhalant allergens: Natural course of sensitization to food and inhalant allergens during the first 6 years of life. *J Allergy Clin Immunol* **103**: 1173–1179.
7. Goh DLM, Chew F-T, Chua K-Y, *et al.* (2000) On bird's nest allergy in Singapore: Edible "bird's nest"-induced anaphylaxis: an under-recognized entity? *J Paeds* **137**: 277–279.
8. Hill DJ, Hosking CS. (2004) On food allergy in young children with eczema: Food allergy and atopic dermatitis in infancy — an epidemiologic study. *Pediatr Allergy Immunol* **15**: 421–427.
9. Høst A, Halken S, Jacobsen HP, *et al.* (2002) On cow's milk allergy in young children: Clinical course of cow's milk protein allergy/intolerance and atopic diseases in childhood. *Peditr Allergy Immunol* **13** (**Suppl. 15**), 23–28.
10. Sampson HA. (2002) On peanut allergy: Peanut allergy. *N Engl J Med* **346**: 1294–1299.

CHAPTER 9: Drug allergy

1. Chowdhury BA. (1999) A reveiw on drug allergy: Drug Reactions. *Cur Pract Med* **2**: *1811–9.*
2. Segal AR, Doherty KM, Leggott J, Zlotoff B. (2007) A nice review on all kind of skin reactions that can be caused by drugs: Cutaneous reactions to drugs in children. *Pediatrics* **120**: 1082–1096.
3. Patterson R, Grammer LC, Greenberger PA, Zeiss CR. (1993) An interesting chapter in a book, on drug allergy: Deswarte RD: Drug allergy. In: *Allergic Diseases and Management* **4th edn,** pp. 395–552. P Lippincott, Philadelphia.
4. Weiss ME. (1992) An overview of drug allergy: Drug allergy. *Med Clin N Am* **28**: 25–8.

5. Aberer W, Bircher A, Romano A, *et al.* (2003) On diagnostic tests for drug allergy: Drug provocation testing in the diagnosis of drug hypersensitivity reactions: general considerations. *Allergy* **58**: 854–63.
6. Lin R. (1992) On penicillin allergy, which is one of the most common drug allergies: A perspective on penicillin allergy. *Arch Int Med* **152**: 930–7.
7. Torres MJ, Mayorga C, Leyva L, *et al.* (2002) Another interesting article to the approach of penicillin allergy: Controlled administration pf penicillin to patients with a positive history but negative skin and specific IgE tests. *Clin Exper Allergy* **32**: 270–6.
8. Baba M, Karakas M, Aksungur VL, *et al.* (2003) On allergy to anti-convulsive drugs: The anticonvulsant hypersensitivity syndrome. *J Eur Acad Derm Vener* **17**: 399–401.
9. Roujeau JC, Stern RS. (1994) On severe reactions to drugs: Severe adverse cutaneous reactions to drugs. *N Engl J Med* **331**: 1272–84.
10. Gruchalla R. (2000) On the mechanisms of drug allergy: Understanding drug allergies. *J Allergy Clin Immunol* **105**: S637–44.

CHAPTER 10: Severe allergic reactions: what can we do?

1. Bock SA, Munoz-Furlong A, Sampson HA. (2001) On severe allergic reactions to foods: Fatalities due to anaphylactic reactions to foods. *J Allergy Clin Immunol* **107**: 191–193.
2. Peavy RD, Metcalfe DD. (2008) On the mechanisms of anaphylaxis: Understanding the mechanisms of anaphylaxis. *Curr Opin Allergy Clin Immunol* **8**: 310–315.
3. El-Shanawany T, Williams PE, Jolles S. (2008) On the approach of the patient with anaphylaxis: Clinical immunology review series — an approach to the patient with anaphylaxis. *Clin Exp Immunol* **153**: 1–9.
4. Bock SA, Muñoz-Furlong A, Sampson HA. (2001) On anaphylaxis to food: Fatalities due to anaphylactic reactions to foods. *J Allergy Clin Immunol* **107**: 191–193.
5. Chiu AM, Kelly KJ. (2005) On the different causes of anaphylaxis: Anaphylaxis: drug allergy, insect stings, and latex. *Immunol Allergy Clin North Am* **25**: 389–405.

6. Järvinen KM, Sicherer SH, Sampson HA, Nowak-Wegrzyn A. (2008) On the treatment of anaphylaxis with epinephrine: Use of multiple doses of epinephrine in food-induced anaphylaxis in children. *J Allergy Clin Immunol* **122**: 133–138
7. Liberman DB, Teach SJ. (2008) On the treatment in children: Management of anaphylaxis in children. *Pediatr Emerg Care* **24**: 861–866.
8. Martelli A, Ghiglioni D, Sarratud T, *et al.* (2008) On the treatment in the emergency room: Anaphylaxis in the emergency department — a paediatric perspective. *Curr Opin Allergy Clin Immunol* **8**: 321–329.
9. Sampson HA. (2003) Another article on the treatment of anaphylaxis: Anaphylaxis and emergency treatment. *Pediatrics* **111**: 1601–1608
10. McKiernan CA, Lieberman SA. (2005) On severe anaphylaxis, leading to shock: Circulatory shock in children — an overview. *Pediatr Rev* **26**: 451–460.

CHAPTER 11: Diagnosis and management of allergic diseases

DIAGNOSIS

1. Wüthrich B. (2005) On the unproven tests and treatments for allergy: Unproven techniques in allergy diagnosis. *J Invest Allergol Clin Immunol* **15**: 86–90.
2. Libeer J-C, Van Hoeyveld E, Kochuyt A-M, *et al.* (2007) On determination of IgE in serum: In vitro determination of allergen-specific serum IgE. Comparative analysis of three methods. *Clin Chem Lab Med* **45**: 413–415.
3. Glovsky MM. (2007) On the evolution of IgE determination: Measuring allergen specific IgE: Where have we been and where are we going now? *Methods Mol Biol* **378**: 205–219.

MANAGEMENT

1. Tovey ER, Almqvist C, Li Q, *et al.* (2008) On early exposure to allergens and its effect on subsequent sensitization: Nonlinear relationship of mite allergen exposure to mite sensitization and asthma in a birth cohort. *J Allergy Clin Immunol* **122**: 114–118.

2. Kalliomäki M, Salminen S, Arvilommi H, *et al.* (2001) The classical study on the prevention of eczema with probiotics: Probiotics in primary prevention of atopic disease: a randomized placebo-controlled trial. *Lancet* **357**: 1076–1079.
3. Taylor AT, Dunstan JA, Prescott SL. (2007) A negative study on the effects of probiotics: Probiotic supplementation for the first 6 months of life fails to reduce the risk of atopic dermatitis and increases the risk of allergen sensitization in high-risk children — a randomized controlled trial. *J Allergy Clin Immunol* **119**: 184–191.
4. Matricardi PM, Björksten B, Bonini S, *et al.* and Wold A for the EAACI Task Force 7. (2003) On the effect of early administration of bacterial products: Microbial products in allergy prevention and therapy. *Allergy* **58**: 461–471.
5. Moro S, Arslanoglu S, Stahl B, *et al.* (2006) On prevention with prebiotics: A mixture of prebiotic oligosaccharides reduces the incidence of atopic dermatitis during the first six months of age. *Arch Dis Childh* **91**: 814–819.
6. Sopo SM, Macchiaiolo M, Zorzi G, Tripodi S. (2004) An overview article on sublingual immunotherapy: Sublingual immunotherapy in asthma and rhinoconjunctivitis — systematic review of paediatric literature. *Arch Dis Childh* **89**: 620–624.
7. Pajno GB, Caminiti L, Vita D, *et al.* (2007) An article on sublingual immunotherapy in children with eczema: Sublingual immunotherapy in mite-sensitized children with atopic dermatitis — a randomized, double-blind, placebo-controlled study. *J Allery Clin Immunol* **120**: 164–170.
8. James LK, Durham SR. (2008) On the mechanisms of immunotherapy: Update on mechanisms of allergen injection immunotherapy. *Clin Exp Allergy* **38**: 1074–1088.
9. Humbert M, Beasley R, Ayres J, *et al.* (2005) On treatment with anti-IgE in severe asthma: Benefits of omalizumab as add-on therapy in patients with severe persistent asthma who are inadequately controlled despite best available therapy (GINA 2002 step 4 treatment) — INNOVATE. *Allergy* **60**: 309–316.
10. Martin-Mateos MA. (2007) On usage of anti-IgE in children: Monoclonal antibodies in pediatrics — use in prevention and treatment. *Allergol Immunopathol* **35**: 145–150.

CHAPTER 12: General Conclusion – The future of allergic diseases in children

1. Martinez FD. (2008) On the genetics of asthma and allergy: Gene-environment interaction in complex diseases — asthma as an illustrative case. *Novartis Found Symp* **293**: 184–192.
2. Lim RH, Kobzik L. (2009) On the genetics of asthma: Maternal transmission of asthma risk. *Am J Reprod Immunol* **61**: 1–10.
3. Kumar R. (2008) On the role of prenatal environment (pregnancy) on allergy: Prenatal factors and the development of asthma. *Curr Opin Pediatr* **20**: 682–687.
4. Sly PD, Boner AL, Björksten B, *et al.* (2008) On early detection of allergy and on primary prevention of allergy: Early identification of atopy in the prediction of persistent asthma in children. *Lancet* **372**: 1100–1106.
5. Hamelmann E, Herz U, Holt P, *et al.* (2008) A review on primary prevention of allergic diseasesNew visions for basic research and primary prevention of pediatric allergy: an IPAC summary and future trends. *Ped Allergy Immunol* **19**: 4–16.
6. Høst A, Halken S, Muraro A, *et al.* (2008) A review on the role of breast feeding and formula feeding in preventing allergy: Dietary prevention of allergic diseases in infants and small children. *Pediatr Allergy Immunol* **19**: 1–4.
7. Sublett JL. (2005) A review of early allergen exposure: The environment and risk factors for atopy. *Curr Allergy Asthma Rep* **5**: 445–450.
8. Thygarajan A, Burks AW. (2008) On the role of early feeding habits and the development of allergy: American Academy of Pediatrics recommendations on the effects of early nutritional interventions on the development of atopic disease. *Curr Opin Pediatr* **20**: 698–702.
9. Vance GH, Holloway JA. (2002) On early contacts with different allergens and its effect on allergy development: Early life exposure to dietary and inhalant allergens. *Pediatr Allergy Immunol* **13 (suppl. 15):** 14–18.
10. Ciaccio CE, Portnoy JM. (2008) On new strategies for primary prevention: Strategies for primary prevention of atopy in children. *Curr Allergy Asthma Rep* **8**: 493–499.

Index

Adrenergic urticaria 153
Adverse food reaction 157, 160
Airway hyperreactivity 72
Allergens xiv, 14, 45, 46, 271, 274
Allergic asthma 55, 74, 77, 78, 126, 256, 257, 260, 261, 276
Allergic March 30, 123, 244, 269
Allergy ii, iii, vi, vii, x, xii, xiv, xvi, xvii, 2, 3, 13–15, 17–21, 23, 27–31, 34–36, 38–43, 46, 47, 49, 50, 52–56, 58, 60–66, 68–70, 73, 74, 76–78, 80–83, 90, 92–95, 97–100, 102, 104, 110, 114, 122–125, 128–131, 133–135, 138, 148, 150, 156–161, 163–165, 167, 169–174, 177, 179–189, 192–194, 199, 200, 202–206, 209, 210, 213, 214, 216, 217, 219, 220, 222, 223, 226–229, 233–235, 238, 240–247, 249, 251, 253–255, 257, 259, 262, 264–272, 275–287
Allergy testing 49, 50, 68, 81, 90, 100, 189, 220, 226–228
Anaphylaxis 12, 28, 29, 42, 55, 64, 67, 68, 143, 150, 153, 164, 170–174, 182, 183, 188, 189, 199, 202, 205, 206, 208, 212–224, 259, 277, 283–285
Anesthetics 155, 189, 205, 206
Angioedema 28, 142, 147, 195

Anti-IgE 235, 244, 260, 261, 286
Antihistamines 98, 101–107, 109, 132, 133, 153–155, 178, 182, 210, 221, 224, 234, 244, 280, 282
Aquagenic urticaria 154
Aspirin 147, 154, 198, 206, 207, 218
Asthma ii, iii, vi, xiv, 19, 21, 25, 37, 38, 72, 73, 79, 80, 83, 85, 183, 184, 241, 261, 274–282, 287
Atopic dermatitis xiv, 22, 46, 110, 116, 141, 145, 148, 149, 162, 231, 254, 277, 280, 281, 283, 286
Atopy 111, 112, 141, 191, 287

Bacterial load 34–36, 39, 251
Bacterial products 134, 253, 254
Beclomethasone dipropionate 86, 105
Beta-agonists 85–88, 210, 244
Beta-lactam antibiotics 67, 189, 190, 201, 202
Biological agents 205
Birch pollen 150, 164, 170
Bird's nest allergy 283
Blomia tropicalis 46, 47, 278
B lymphocytes 4, 6, 9, 16
Bone marrow 5, 6, 10, 11
Breast feeding 78, 265, 287
Bronchial asthma 72, 74, 75, 85, 97
Budesonide 86, 105, 210

Cap 176, 178, 236, 241
Casein 62
Cat allergy 54, 55
Celiac disease 64, 167, 168
Cetirizine 103, 104, 153, 154, 233, 234
Cholinergic urticaria 153, 154
Cockroach allergy 52, 66
Conjunctivitis 19, 23, 39, 81, 92, 93, 95, 99, 100, 106, 108, 109, 163, 197, 259, 280
Corticosteroids 85, 86, 88, 101, 102, 105–107, 109, 153, 155, 166, 182, 197, 198, 210, 221, 244, 250, 257, 261, 280
Cow's milk allergy 62, 254, 283

Dendritic cells 7, 10, 11, 258, 276
Dermatophagoides farinae 15, 46, 47, 50, 51
Dermatophagoides pteronyssinus 46, 47
Dermographism 152, 232, 282
Desloratidine 103, 105, 154
Diet 43, 62, 79, 166, 167, 172, 173, 175, 176, 179, 182, 242, 243, 247
Disodium cromoglycate 101, 109
Dog allergy 55
Double-blind placebo-controlled food challenge (dbpcfc) 179
Drug allergy 46, 68, 186–189, 192, 193, 199, 200, 209, 210, 233, 234, 277, 283, 284

Eczema vii, xii, xiv, xv, 3, 4, 9, 13, 19–22, 26, 30, 31, 35, 37–39, 41, 43, 44, 52, 55, 59, 62–64, 77, 81, 102, 103, 106, 145, 148, 157, 160, 163, 166, 169, 174, 176, 179, 190, 230, 233, 235, 240, 244–246, 250, 253, 254, 259, 261, 264, 265, 269, 277, 280, 281, 283, 286
Eczema herpeticum 26
Egg allergy 41, 62, 63, 205, 282
Eosinophil 10
Eosinophilic gastroenteritis 165, 166
Epidemiology xvi, 32–34, 37, 39, 41, 61, 157, 173, 189, 213, 270, 276, 277
Epinephrine 155, 182, 183, 209, 210, 220–224, 257, 285
Epipen 28, 155, 182, 210, 220, 221, 224, 233
Erythema multiforme 144, 196, 197

Fish allergy 42, 43, 65, 66, 172, 173, 246, 247
Fluticasone 86, 105
Food additives 41, 147–149, 241
Food allergy vii, 15, 28–30, 39–41, 43, 50, 62, 63, 65, 66, 77, 156–161, 163, 169–171, 173, 174, 177, 179–183, 188, 213, 214, 233, 234, 254, 259, 265, 269, 271, 272, 275, 277, 282, 283
Food aversion 158, 160
Food intolerance 158

Ger = gastroesophageal reflux 79
Granulocytes 6, 9

Hamster allergy 55
Hapten 14, 67, 190, 191
Histamine 4, 12, 17, 29, 82, 102, 145, 146, 152, 158, 161, 176, 178, 188, 208, 209, 218, 229–231, 249
Holistic approach 83
House dust mites xiv, xvi, 14, 15, 21, 30, 40, 43, 45, 46, 48–50, 52, 55, 61, 66, 72, 80, 92, 94, 95, 102, 106, 173, 174, 227, 233, 245, 247–249, 251, 256, 259, 265, 269, 271
Hydrolyzed formula 265
Hygiene hypothesis 34, 251, 276
Hypersensitivity syndrome 195, 197, 284

Immune response 3, 5, 7, 10–13, 44, 162, 190, 192, 258
Immune system 2, 3, 5–8, 10, 15, 16, 26, 35, 158, 167, 169, 180, 182, 187, 188, 212, 232, 248, 251, 252, 255, 264, 276

Immunotherapy vii, 53, 65, 83, 85, 91, 101, 106, 109, 147, 150, 182, 227, 234, 244, 255–259, 264, 267, 270, 272, 274, 277, 286
Incidence xi, 32, 33, 67, 141, 143, 189, 201, 204, 208, 214, 245, 265, 286
Inflammation 3, 4, 12, 15, 17, 20, 21, 23, 24, 39, 44, 72, 73, 75, 76, 78, 82, 86, 95, 98, 105, 144, 221, 250, 276
Inhaled corticosteroids 86, 261
Inhalers 103
Insect bites 29, 144, 147, 150, 219
Insulin 189, 190, 204, 209, 217
Interleukins 5, 12
Intradermal test 178, 243
Intranasal corticosteroids 101, 102, 105, 106, 280

Latex allergy 69, 70, 150, 164, 282
Levocetirizine 103, 104, 154
Loratadine 103, 104, 154
Lung function testing 81, 82, 90
Lyell syndrome 195, 197, 204
Lymph nodes 7, 9, 11, 194
Lymphocytes 4–7, 9, 12, 16, 160, 162, 191, 199, 256, 276

Macrophages 7, 10, 12, 16, 258, 276
Mast cell 4, 11, 15, 16, 145, 146, 148, 152, 153, 218, 229–231, 250, 276
Molluscum contagiosum 26
Montelukast 86, 101, 106
Morbidity ii, 33, 58, 93, 108, 186, 194, 196–198, 201, 262
Mortality 33, 186, 196, 197, 204, 214

Natural killer cells 7, 9, 12
Non-steroidal anti-inflammatory drugs (NSAIDS) 189

Omalizumab (anti-IGE) 260
Oral allergy syndrome (oas) 164, 165, 170
Otitis media 20, 24, 97
Ovalbumine 63, 205

Paracetamol 35, 188, 189, 207, 208
Peanut allergy 42, 64, 65, 148, 172, 173, 272, 283
Penicillin 14, 28, 46, 67, 68, 147, 189, 191–193, 201–203, 209, 210, 215, 217, 284
Physical urticaria 27, 143, 147, 151–153
Pollen xiv, 14, 45, 52, 58–61, 64, 72, 80, 94, 95, 102, 106, 150, 151, 164, 165, 170, 171, 181, 216, 232, 233, 245, 247, 249, 256, 257, 259, 269, 278

Pollution 33, 36, 53, 72, 78–80, 249, 265, 266
Prebiotics 251–253, 266, 267, 286
Pressure-induced urticaria 152
Prevalence ii, xi, 32, 33, 35, 37–41, 43, 52, 54, 66, 73, 76, 93, 147, 157, 171–174, 189, 193, 213, 214, 246, 247, 262, 267, 270, 277, 278, 282
Primary prevention of allergy 269, 287
Probiotics 35, 251–254, 266, 267, 286
Prognosis ii, 74, 82, 85, 91, 180, 181, 209, 257, 279
Protein 3, 9, 14, 41, 45, 55, 62, 64, 66, 148, 167, 190, 195, 229, 278, 283
Provocation test 200, 203, 228, 242
Pruritus 143–145, 204, 209, 215

Rast 176, 178, 236, 241
Regulatory t cell 7, 13, 276
Reliever medication 88
Rhinitis vii, xii, xiii, xiv, 3, 4, 12, 19, 20–25, 28, 30, 31, 35, 37–39, 43, 44, 46, 52, 55, 59, 69, 79, 81, 85, 92, 93, 94–101, 107, 163–165, 169, 206, 215, 233, 240, 244, 245, 250, 253, 254, 256, 257, 259, 268, 270, 279, 280, 282
Rhino-sinusitis 24, 79, 80, 92, 95–97, 99, 100, 107, 108, 261, 270

Scabies 138, 139, 144
Seborrhoeic eczema 110, 136, 137
Serum sickness 147, 195, 199, 201
Sinusitis 20, 24, 25, 74, 79, 80, 85, 92, 95–97, 99, 100, 107, 108, 206, 261, 270, 280
Skin prick testing (spt) 176, 199, 228
Solar urticaria 154
Soy allergy 64, 180
Spleen 5, 7, 9, 11
Staphylococcus aureus 26, 117, 119, 130, 138
Stevens-johnson syndrome 195–197, 200, 210
Subcutaneous immunotherapy 91, 255, 256
Sublingual immunotherapy (SLIT) 101, 182, 255–257
Sulfonamides 189, 191, 195, 198, 204
Synbiotics 101, 134, 251–253, 266, 267

Tacrolimus 132–134
Thymus 5, 6, 11
T lymphocytes 6, 7, 16, 276

Tobacco smoke 78
Toxic Epidermal Necrolysis (Lyell syndrome) 195, 204
Tree nut allergy 65

Urticaria xiv, xv, 12, 19, 27, 28, 31, 41, 44, 50, 51, 55, 56, 59, 63, 64, 69, 80, 103, 124, 131, 140–155, 157, 162–165, 169, 174, 193, 194, 201, 204, 206–208, 214, 215, 219, 226, 233, 257, 281, 282
Urticarial lesions 141

Vasculitis 144, 147, 193, 194, 195

Warts 26, 117, 120–121
Wheat allergy 64
Wheezing xiv, 21, 39, 73–75, 81, 88, 90, 91, 163, 164, 214, 215, 250, 274, 278, 279